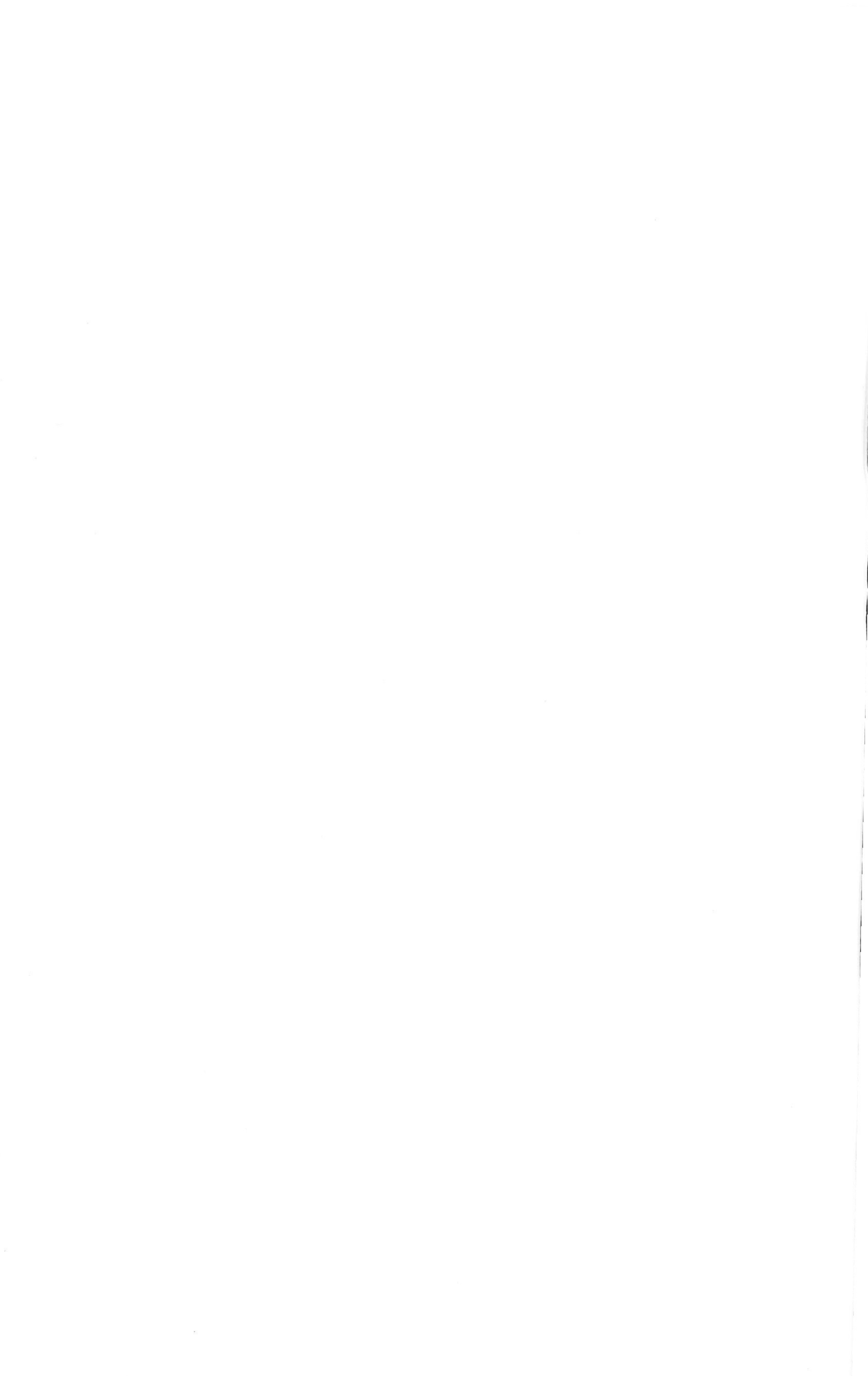

Vascular Anesthesia

Editor

CHARLES C. HILL

ANESTHESIOLOGY CLINICS

www.anesthesiology.theclinics.com

Consulting Editor
LEE A. FLEISHER

September 2014 • Volume 32 • Number 3

ELSEVIER

1600 John F. Kennedy Boulevard • Suite 1800 • Philadelphia, Pennsylvania, 19103-2899

http://www.theclinics.com

ANESTHESIOLOGY CLINICS Volume 32, Number 3
September 2014 ISSN 1932-2275, ISBN-13: 978-0-323-32311-6

Editor: Jennifer Flynn-Briggs
Developmental Editor: Susan Showalter

Anesthesiology Clinics (ISSN 1932-2275) is published quarterly by Elsevier Inc., 360 Park Avenue South, New York, NY 10010-1710. Months of issue are March, June, September, and December. Periodicals postage paid at New York, NY and at additional mailing offices. Subscription prices are $160.00 per year (US student/resident), $330.00 per year (US individuals), $400.00 per year (Canadian individuals), $533.00 per year (US institutions), $674.00 per year (Canadian institutions), $225.00 per year (Canadian and foreign student/resident), $455.00 per year (foreign individuals), and $674.00 per year (foreign institutions). To receive student and resident rate, orders must be accompanied by name of affiliated institution, date of term, and the *signature* of program/residency coordinator on institutions letterhead. Orders will be billed at individual rate until proof of status is received. Foreign air speed delivery is included in all *Clinics'* subscription prices. All prices are subject to change without notice. POSTMASTER: Send address changes to *Anesthesiology Clinics,* Elsevier Health Sciences Division, Subscription Customer Service, 3251 Riverport Lane, Maryland Heights, MO 63043. Customer Service (orders, claims, online, change of address): Elsevier Health Sciences Division, Subscription Customer Service, 3251 Riverport Lane, Maryland Heights, MO 63043. Tel:1-800-654-2452 (U.S. and Canada); 314-447-8871 (outside U.S. and Canada). Fax: 314-447-8029. E-mail: journalscustomerservice-usa@elsevier.com (for print support); journalsonlinesupport-usa@elsevier.com (for online support).

Reprints. For copies of 100 or more of articles in this publication, please contact the Commercial Reprints Department, Elsevier Inc., 360 Park Avenue South, New York, NY 10010-1710. Tel.: 212-633-3874; Fax: 212-633-3820; E-mail: reprints@elsevier.com.

Anesthesiology Clinics, is also published in Spanish by McGraw-Hill Inter-americana Editores S. A., P.O. Box 5-237, 06500 Mexico D. F., Mexico.

Anesthesiology Clinics, is covered in *MEDLINE/PubMed (Index Medicus), Current Contents/Clinical Medicine, Excerpta Medica, ISI/BIOMED*, and *Chemical Abstracts*.

Contributors

CONSULTING EDITOR

LEE A. FLEISHER, MD
Robert D. Dripps Professor and Chair of Anesthesiology and Critical Care, Professor of Medicine, Perelman School of Medicine, University of Pennsylvania, Philadelphia, Pennsylvania

EDITOR

CHARLES C. HILL, MD
Clinical Assistant Professor, Medical Director Cardiovascular ICU, Department of Anesthesiology, Perioperative and Pain Medicine, Stanford University Medical Center, Stanford University School of Medicine, Stanford, California

AUTHORS

JAMES M. ANTON, MD
Assistant Professor and Associate Chief of Anesthesia, St. Luke's Medical Group, CHI St. Luke's Health; Fellowship Program Director, Division of Cardiovascular Anesthesiology, Texas Heart Institute, Baylor St. Luke's Medical Center, Houston, Texas

ANDREY APINIS, MD
Assistant Professor, Cardiothoracic Anesthesiology, Montefiore Medical Center, Albert Einstein College of Medicine, Bronx, New York

ETTORE CRIMI, MD
Clinical Assistant Professor, Department of Anesthesia and Critical Care Medicine, Shands Hospital, University of Florida, Gainesville, Florida

RYAN DERBY, MD, MPH
Clinical Assistant Professor, Stanford Hospital and Clinics, Stanford, California

KENNETH D. EICHENBAUM, MD, MSE
Fellow, Division of Cardiothoracic Anesthesia, Department of Anesthesiology, Perioperative and Pain Medicine, Stanford University Medical Center, Stanford, California

JAMES FLAHERTY, MD
Resident, Stanford Hospital and Clinics, Stanford, California

KATHERINE GRICHNIK, MD
American Anesthesiology, Mednax National Medical Group, Sunrise, Florida

CHARLES C. HILL, MD
Clinical Assistant Professor, Medical Director Cardiovascular ICU, Department of Anesthesiology, Perioperative and Pain Medicine, Stanford University Medical Center, Stanford University School of Medicine, Stanford, California

JEAN-LOUIS HORN, MD
Professor, Stanford Hospital and Clinics, Stanford, California

JASON T. LEE, MD
Division of Vascular Surgery, Stanford University Medical Center, Stanford, California

JONATHAN LEFF, MD
Chief, Cardiothoracic Anesthesiology; Director Cardiothoracic Anesthesia Fellowship, Associate Professor, Montefiore Medical Center, Albert Einstein College of Medicine, Bronx, New York

YASDET MALDONADO, MD
Department of Anesthesiology, Allegheny Health Network, Temple University School of Medicine, Pittsburgh, Pennsylvania

MARIE LAPENTA MCHENRY, MD
Chief Resident, Department of Anesthesiology, Perioperative and Pain Medicine, Stanford Hospital and Clinics, Stanford, California

DARYL A. OAKES, MD
Clinical Assistant Professor, Division of Cardiothoracic Anesthesia, Department of Anesthesiology, Perioperative and Pain Medicine, Stanford University Medical Center, Stanford, California

STEPHEN SAMS, MD
Department of Anesthesiology, Beaumont Health System, Royal Oak, Michigan

SANKALP SEHGAL, MD
Fellow, Cardiothoracic Anesthesiology, Montefiore Medical Center, Albert Einstein College of Medicine, Bronx, New York

SAKET SINGH, MD
Department of Anesthesiology, Allegheny Health Network, Temple University School of Medicine, Pittsburgh, Pennsylvania

ROY SOTO, MD
Department of Anesthesiology, Beaumont Health System, Royal Oak, Michigan; American Anesthesiology, Mednax National Medical Group, Sunrise, Florida

MARK A. TAYLOR, MD
Department of Anesthesiology, Allegheny Health Network, Temple University School of Medicine, Pittsburgh, Pennsylvania

BRANT W. ULLERY, MD
Division of Vascular Surgery, Stanford University Medical Center, Stanford, California

Contents

ANESTHESIOLOGY CLINICS

FORTHCOMING ISSUES

December 2014
Orthopedic Anesthesia
Nabil Elkassabany and
Edward Mariano, *Editors*

March 2015
Anesthetic Care for Abdominal Surgery
Timothy Miller and
Michael Scott, *Editors*

RECENT ISSUES

June 2014
Ambulatory Anesthesiology
Jeffrey L. Apfelbaum
and Thomas W. Cutter, *Editors*

March 2014
Pediatric Anesthesiology
Alan Jay Schwartz, Dean B. Andropoulos,
and Andrew Davidson, *Editors*

December 2013
Abdominal Transplantation
Claus U. Niemann, *Editor*

September 2013
Obstetric Anesthesia
Robert Gaiser, *Editor*

RELATED INTEREST

Cardiology Clinics, November 2013 (Volume 31, Issue 4)
Cardiovascular Intensive Care
Umesh K. Gidwani, Samin K. Sharma, and Annapoorna S. Kini, *Editors*

Foreword

Vascular Anesthesia

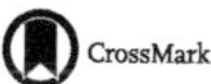

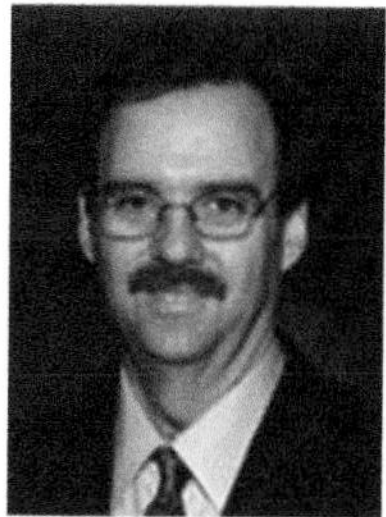

Lee A. Fleisher, MD
Consulting Editor

Given the prevalence of atherosclerosis, peripheral vascular disease continues to require surgical interventions. Despite numerous advances in interventional and less invasive techniques, many of these patients still require an anesthetic. In this issue of *Anesthesiology Clinics*, a group of experts in the care of these patients outlined management from the preoperative evaluation to postoperative care. In addition, there is an excellent article on surgical care, which is critical for providing optimal anesthesia for our patients.

In choosing a guest editor for this issue, I solicited Charles Hill, MD, Clinical Assistant Professor at Stanford University. Charles completed a residency in Anesthesiology at Vanderbilt University Medical Center and a Fellowship in Cardiovascular Anesthesiology at Stanford University Medical. He subsequently joined the faculty, where he is Medical Director of the Cardiovascular ICU. For this topic, he has brought together experts to help inform our practice.

Lee A. Fleisher, MD
Perelman School of Medicine
University of Pennsylvania
Philadelphia, PA 19104, USA

E-mail address:
lee.fleisher@uphs.upenn.edu

Anesthesiology Clin 32 (2014) ix
http://dx.doi.org/10.1016/j.anclin.2014.07.001 anesthesiology.theclinics.com
1932-2275/14/$ – see front matter

Preface

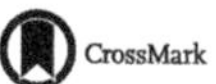

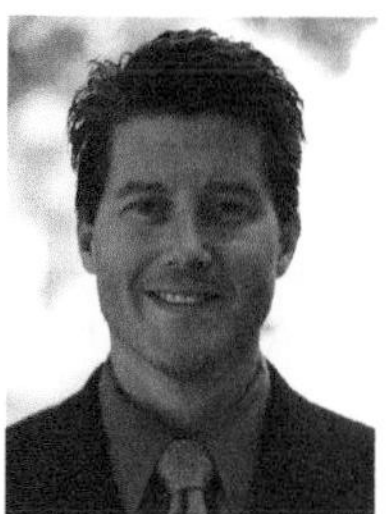

Charles C. Hill, MD
Editor

The perioperative care of vascular surgery patients, is an increasingly complex and challenging task for anesthesiologists. These patients are often elderly, frail and suffering from multiple chronic disease states. Their comorbidities frequently dominate their perioperative medical course and remain prominent in their postoperative medical care. Accordingly, these high-risk patients require appropriate patient selection and preoperative medical optimization. Meticulous intraoperative anesthetic management followed by experienced and diligent postoperative care helps mitigate end-organ ischemia and ensure successful outcomes.

This issue of *Anesthesiology Clinics* is devoted to the perioperative medical and surgical management of the patient presenting with vascular disease. We have examined the full spectrum of care for these patients, beginning with the preoperative evaluation and continuing through the critical care considerations following all of the major vascular surgical procedures. We also discusses the optimal medical management of these complicated patients, with a focus on the recent literature that will serve as an evidence-based framework for the future clinical treatment of these patients.

Specific areas of clinical concern related to the anesthetic and surgical management of the vascular patient are examined in detail. Regional anesthesia and its importance to the safe and efficient management of the vascular surgical patient is described, including an overview of the regional techniques frequently associated with vascular surgical procedures. The perioperative management of lower extremity revascularization is reviewed, along with a discussion of the significant comorbidities encountered in this patient population. Evolving intraoperative anesthetic management concepts are examined for both carotid endarterectomy and combined coronary artery bypass grafting and carotid endarterectomy. This issue also presents a surgical perspective on the modern-day management of complex abdominal aneurysms.

Anesthesiology Clin 32 (2014) xi–xii
http://dx.doi.org/10.1016/j.anclin.2014.06.001 anesthesiology.theclinics.com
1932-2275/14/$ – see front matter

We hope you find this edition of *Anesthesiology Clinics* educational and enjoyable. Thank you for the privilege to facilitate the care of your vascular surgery patients.

Charles C. Hill, MD
Cardiovascular ICU
Department of Anesthesiology, Perioperative and Pain Medicine
Stanford University
300 Pasteur Drive
Stanford, CA 9305, USA

E-mail address:
chill1@stanford.edu

Preoperative Evaluation of the Vascular Surgery Patient

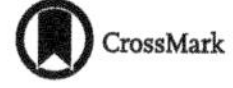

Stephen Sams, MD[a], Katherine Grichnik, MD[b], Roy Soto, MD[a,b,*]

KEYWORDS

• Vascular surgery • Preoperative evaluation • Endovascular • Cardiac clearance • Contrast nephropathy

KEY POINTS

- Patients requiring vascular surgery are complex with multiple comorbidities.
- Minimally invasive surgical techniques allow procedures to be done in high-risk patients.
- Vascular surgical procedures are ever evolving with variable intraoperative management concerns that should be considered in the preoperative assessment.
- Risk assessment for perioperative morbidity and mortality should seek variables that can be improved before surgery.

INTRODUCTION

Patients requiring vascular surgery present a multitude of perioperative challenges due to increasingly complex comorbidities in an ever-aging patient population. This, coupled with less-invasive surgical techniques that allow more patients to be considered "acceptable" surgical candidates, creates the need for effective preoperative anesthetic evaluations.

Patients requiring vascular surgery often have preexisting cardiovascular, pulmonary, renal, and endocrine dysfunction, and it is not surprising that morbidity is higher, and long-term survival is lower than for patients having nonvascular procedures. Some of these comorbidities may not have been recognized or have been poorly managed at the time of surgical presentation. Feringa and colleagues[1] noted that unrecognized myocardial infarction and silent myocardial ischemia were detected in

---

Disclosure Statement: No authors report a current or previous relationship between themselves and any company or organization with a vested interest in the outcome of this study.
[a] Department of Anesthesiology, Beaumont Health System, 3601 West 13-Mile Road, Royal Oak, MI 48073, USA; [b] American Anesthesiology, Mednax National Medical Group, 1301 Concord Terrace, Sunrise, FL 33322, USA
* Corresponding author. Department of Anesthesiology, Beaumont Health System, 3601 West 13-Mile Road, Royal Oak, MI 48073.
E-mail address: roy.soto@beaumont.edu

Anesthesiology Clin 32 (2014) 599–614
http://dx.doi.org/10.1016/j.anclin.2014.05.006 anesthesiology.theclinics.com
1932-2275/14/$ – see front matter

23% and 28%, respectively, of vascular surgery patients studied; these patients had a worse survival compared with patients with no symptoms or signs of coronary artery disease (CAD).

Layered on the baseline patient characteristics are the complexity and challenges inherent to the various vascular procedures themselves. The anesthesia care team must not only have a firm grasp of concurrent disease processes, but also must be familiar with the particular surgical procedure and integrate the consequences of the surgical procedure on baseline disease. Further, the introduction of endovascular surgical techniques changed the specific needs of intraoperative anesthetic care. For example, endovascular repair of abdominal aortic aneurysms (AAA) has surpassed open repair across all age groups,[2] eliminating the consequences of prolonged aortic clamping, but introducing the need for new monitoring and evaluation strategies.

This review uses a systems-based approach to presurgical patient evaluation, followed by a discussion of the anesthetic implications of specific vascular procedures and overall risk.

SYSTEMS-BASED PREOPERATIVE EVALUATION

Cardiovascular Assessment

Patients with vascular disease frequently suffer from concurrent cardiac disease. As a result, cardiac evaluation and optimization are a primary component of preoperative assessment. Standard preoperative cardiac assessment includes an appraisal of baseline health status, exercise tolerance, and electrocardiogram (ECG) analysis. Abnormal findings on history or ECG should prompt further noninvasive cardiac testing to assess the response to exercise, as well as an estimate of ventricular reserve and myocardium at risk. Testing must be coordinated with cardiology and may include routine treadmill assessment, stress echocardiography, and nucleotide studies.

Abnormal findings on these tests may result in percutaneous interventions and/or coronary revascularization, but the degree of testing and subsequent intervention must be balanced against the level of proposed surgical insult. For example, patients undergoing arterial-venous graft revision or percutaneous lower-extremity procedures may incur less intraoperative physiologic trespass than an open AAA or carotid artery repair, despite the high risk for perioperative complications. A risk/benefit analysis also must be considered with the preoperative evaluation to assess whether a particular test will alter the approach to patient care.

This methodology is supported by the American College of Cardiology (ACC) and American Heart Association (AHA) recommendations, which include the suggestion that preoperative cardiac testing should be considered only if the results would impact the proposed anesthetic and surgical management plan.[3] Using the updated 2007 ACC/AHA recommendations and their recent meta-analysis, Omar and colleagues developed useful and practical algorithms for preoperative cardiac assessment before vascular surgery for (1) patients with stable or asymptomatic CAD and (2) patients with CAD (**Figs. 1** and **2**).

It is particularly important to elicit a history of coronary stent placement in the vascular surgical population. There is a high incidence of morbidity and mortality associated with surgical procedures being performed within 6 months of stent placement, and with premature cessation of antiplatelet therapy resulting in in-stent thrombosis. Current guidelines recommend the following: (1) elective surgery after drug-eluting stent (DES) implantation should be delayed until completion of 1 year of dual antiplatelet therapy, and (2) if surgery is urgent, it should be performed without cessation of antiplatelet therapy.[4]

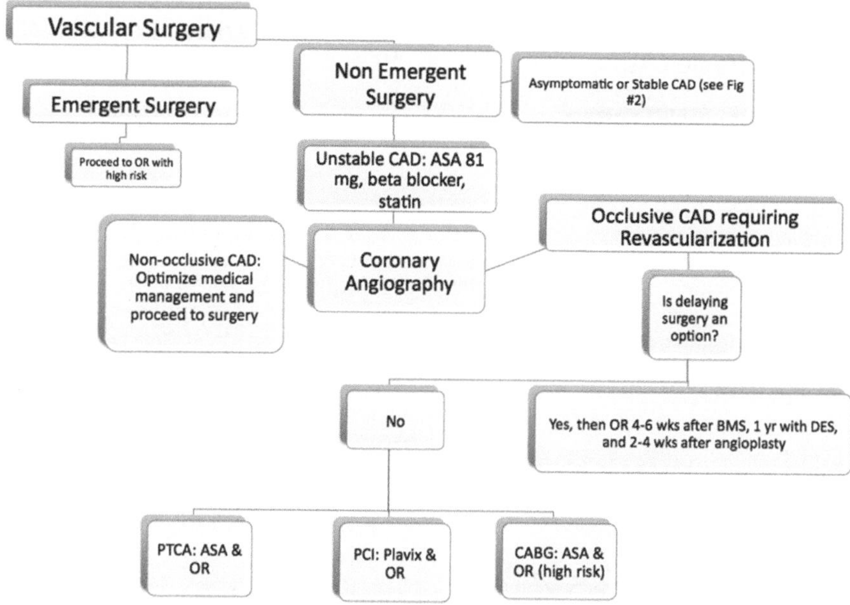

Fig. 1. Preoperative cardiac evaluation for patients with asymptomatic or stable CAD. ASA, acetylsalicylic acid; BMS, bare-metal stent; CABG, coronary artery bypass grafting; OR, operating room; PCI, percutaneous coronary intervention; PTCA, percutaneous transluminal coronary angioplasty; wks, weeks. (*Data from* Omar HR, Mangar D, Camporesi EM. Preoperative cardiac evaluation of the vascular surgery patient—an anesthesia perspective. Vasc Endovascular Surg 2012;46(3):201–11.)

The guidelines for DES differ from those for bare-metal stents, with the recommendation to delay surgery and temporary cessation of antiplatelet drugs for only 4 to 6 weeks after stent placement.[3] Of note, a recent analysis challenges these guidelines and states that major adverse cardiac events with noncardiac surgery were associated with emergency surgery and advanced cardiac disease but not stent type or timing of surgery beyond 6 months after stent implantation.[5]

Intriguingly, some evidence suggests that risk for postoperative complications, especially adverse cardiac events, may be predicted by preoperative testing of markers of inflammation. Common preoperative biomarkers that can be easily tested include C-reactive protein, brain natriuretic peptide (BNP) concentration, and troponin I. Of these, BNP seems to be the most valuable for overall risk prediction. Preoperative BNP elevation is associated with myocardium at risk and is an independent predictor of adverse cardiac events.[6] Further, preoperative BNP levels below a certain threshold have been shown to identify patients who have a lower risk of cardiac complications after vascular surgery.[7]

In elective vascular surgical procedures, Biccard and colleagues[8] demonstrated that preoperative troponin and BNP levels could influence risk prediction through reclassification of patients into “higher” or “lower” risk categories, with the goal of optimizing clinical management. However, they found that, although measurement of troponins guided overall patient risk reclassification, a subset of patients who experienced a major adverse event had been reclassified as “low” risk. Thus troponins alone should not be used to exclude patients from a higher-risk category. In contrast, preoperative BNP levels were very useful for risk stratification as an independent predictor of major harmful cardiac events.

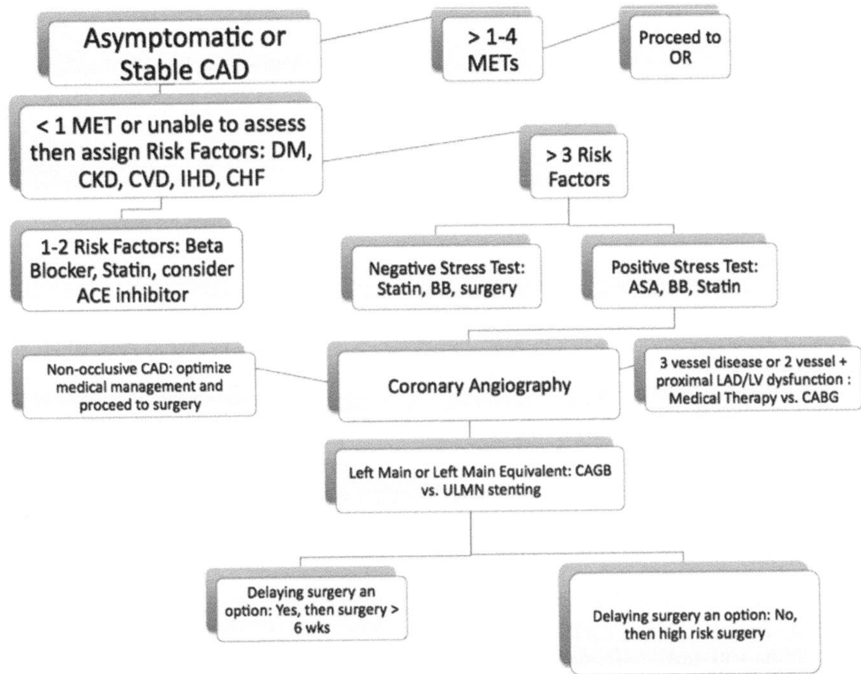

Fig. 2. Preoperative cardiac evaluation for patients with unstable CAD or major vascular surgery. ACE, angiotensin-converting enzyme; ASA, acetylsalicylic acid; BB, beta blocker; CABG, coronary artery bypass grafting; CHF, congestive heart failure; CKD, chronic kidney disease; CVD, cerebrovascular disease; DM, diabetes mellitus; IHD, ischemic heart disease; LAD/LV, left anterior descending/left ventricle; METs, metabolic equivalents; OR, operating room; ULMN, unprotected left main. (*Data from* Omar HR, Mangar D, Camporesi EM. Preoperative cardiac evaluation of the vascular surgery patient—an anesthesia perspective. Vasc Endovascular Surg 2012;46(3):201–11.)

Cardiovascular Medications

Preoperative medication management for patients with cardiac and vascular disease also has been an active area of controversy over the past decade. Beta-blockers have been a focus of much of this controversy, with the prior recommendations for near-universal treatment of vascular surgical patients now revised. The ACC/AHA 2009 update on perioperative cardiovascular evaluation recommends specifically limiting beta-blocker treatment to those on preexisting beta-blocker therapy or those who have been found to have reversible ischemia on preoperative testing.[9]

Indeed, the introduction of preoperative beta blockade in a beta-blocker–naïve patient has been shown to increase perioperative risk. The 2008 PeriOperative ISchemic Evaluation (POISE) trial, which investigated the effect of starting metoprolol on beta-blocker–naïve patients 2 to 4 hours before noncardiac surgery, showed increased cardiovascular and total mortality. The reasons for this increase in morbidity and mortality resulted from increased nonfatal stroke, clinically significant hypotension, and severe bradycardia.[10,11] Recommendations for beta-blocker therapy have been challenged and are likely to change in the future.[12] However, quality-of-care metrics are using the most currently available guidelines, as stated previously.

Patients with vascular disease also are often prescribed anticoagulants for cardiac and vascular conditions.[13] Medications range from the simple (aspirin) to the complex (the novel oral anticoagulants: direct Factor Xa or IIa inhibitors). Each medication carries its own unique risks and challenges, especially relating to reversibility and timing of cessation before surgery (**Table 1**). Importantly, several anticoagulants have no specific reversal agent, which can pose a challenge in the face of a planned regional anesthetic, or with surgical bleeding.[14,15]

For elective procedures, the first consideration is whether there is a need to bridge the patient to low molecular weight heparin after cessation of the oral agent.[16] This decision is dictated by the calculated risk of an adverse event from the underlying condition in the absence of anticoagulation. For example, a patient being treated with rivaroxaban for atrial fibrillation with a $CHADS_2$ score (**Table 2**) of 4 may need a bridging anticoagulant to prevent stroke before surgery. It is advisable to consult with the patient's primary care provider or cardiologist for bridging therapy.

A second consideration is the timing of oral anticoagulant cessation before surgery, which is especially important in the absence of both a reversal agent and an effective test of anticoagulation for the direct Factor Xa or IIa inhibitors. As direct Factor Xa or IIa inhibitors have recently been widely approved, there are no firm guidelines based on experience. It is reasonable to allow these drugs to dissipate in accordance with their half-life and a conservative approach would be to allow a drug to clear for 5 half-lives from drug cessation. However, others advocate for shorter periods of cessation (see **Table 1**).

Equally important is the resumption of an oral anticoagulant after surgery. The onset of the direct Factor Xa or IIa inhibitors is rapid, and catheter-based neuraxial analgesics are contraindicated with these drugs. It is important to understand these risks and challenges, especially if neuraxial regional analgesia is being considered.[17]

Antiplatelet agents, primarily used to prevent embolic events, may be used in concurrence with anticoagulants, which are primarily used to prevent thrombotic events. Thus, patients with carotid or peripheral vascular disease, as well as those with coronary or other vascular stents, are likely to be treated with an antiplatelet agent. Similarly, the need to discontinue an agent before surgery must be weighed against the risk of an embolic event; consultation with the patient's primary care provider or cardiologist is advised to determine the correct management strategy for an individual patient. Of note, most will continue aspirin but withhold other antiplatelet agents, such as clopidogrel, before elective surgery.

Intriguing evidence suggests that preoperative statin therapy also may play a role in optimizing care in this patient population. The initiation of statin therapy in patients undergoing vascular surgery has been shown to decrease myocardial ischemia during and shortly after surgery, as well as decrease postoperative mortality related to cardiovascular events.[18] These beneficial effects are attributed to the ability of statins to improve endothelial function, stabilize atherosclerotic plaques, and reduce oxidative stress, culminating in an overall state of decreased vascular inflammation.[19]

In addition to cardiovascular benefits, initiating statin therapy before vascular surgery has other benefits. Preoperative statin use is associated with stable or improved renal function by evidence of reduced incidence of postoperative renal insufficiency and earlier recovery of kidney dysfunction after endovascular procedures.[20,21] Recommendations for dosage and type of statin in vascular patients include at least 20 mg per day of either atorvastatin or rosuvastatin.[22] Evidence also suggests that statins be started a minimum of 2 weeks before elective vascular procedures and continued throughout the preoperative period.[23] Routine initiation of statin therapy should therefore be strongly considered for all patients undergoing vascular procedures, with special consideration being given to timing of the procedure.[24]

Table 1
Anticoagulant and antiplatelet agents commonly used in vascular surgical patients

	ASA/NSAIDs	Clopidogrel	Warfarin	Fondaparinux	Enoxaparin	Edoxaban	Apixaban	Rivaroxaban	Dabigatran
Mechanism of action	COX inhibitor	ADP-GPIIb/IIIa complex inhibitor	Inhibits factor II, VII, IX, X, protein C and S	Binds antithrombin III and inhibits FXa	Anti FXa and Anti FIIa	Anti FXa	Direct FXa inhibitor	Direct FXa inhibitor	Direct thrombin inhibitor
Dosing	Oral	Oral	Oral	SQ	SQ	Oral	Oral BID	Oral QD	Oral BID
Peak concentration after administration, h	0.5–1.0	0.5–1.0	4	1–3	3–5	1–2	1–3	1–4	1–2
Half-life, h	6	6	20–60	17–21	4–7	9–11	8–15	10	12–17
Metabolism/ elimination	Hepatic/ renal	Hepatic/ renal and fecal	Hepatic/ primarily renal	Primarily renal	Hepatic/ primarily renal	Renal ~50%	Liver ~70%/ Renal ~30%	Hepatic/ Renal ~66%	Renal ~80%
Routine monitoring assay	None. Bleeding time prolonged.	None.	Frequent INR/PT.	None. Anti-FXa levels in select patients.	None. Anti-FXa levels in select patients.	None.	None. PT some correlation.	None specifically. PT some correlation.	None specifically. PT, INR, aPTT, TT, ECT prolonged.

Antidote and reversal agents	No specific antidote. Consider platelets.	No specific antidote. Consider blood products.	FFP, and other factor concentrates/ vitamin K.	None specifically, rFVIIA may be effective.	Protamine and blood products.	No specific antidote. Consider charcoal within 2–6 h. Possible recombinant FVIIA, APCC, PCC.	No specific antidote. Consider charcoal within 2–6 h. Possible recombinant FVIIA, APCC, PCC.	No specific antidote. FFP may not be effective. Charcoal within 2 h. Possible recombinant FVIIA, APCC, PCC.	No specific antidote. Consider charcoal if within 1–2 h. Possible recombinant FVIIA, FEIBA, APCC, PCC.
Hemodialysis	Dialyzable.	Unlikely, inconclusive	Not effective.	Not effective.	Not effective.	Not effective.	Not effective.	Not effective.	60% dialyzable.
When to stop (no. of days preop) or with regard to neuraxial procedures	Variable or may be given.	Consult with cardiologist, usually 7 d.	Until INR normalized.	48 h before neuraxial procedure.	12 h before neuraxial procedure.	5–7 d for high risk bleeding operations. Neuraxial: None official, 45–55 h.	5–7 d for high risk bleeding operations. Neuraxial: None official, 60 h.	5 d for high-risk bleeding operations. Neuraxial: None official, some state 18–24 h, others 35–55 h.	5–7 d for high-risk bleeding operations. Neuraxial: None official, 60–85 h.

Abbreviations: APCC, activated prothrombin complex concentrates; aPTT, activated partial thromboplastin time; ASA, acetylsalicylic acid; ECT, ecarin clotting time; FEIBA, factor eight inhibitor bypassing activity; FFP, fresh frozen plasma; INR, international normalized ratio; SQ, subcutaneous; TT, thrombin time.

Table 2
CHADS$_2$ risk assessment and treatment plan for patients with atrial fibrillation

CHADS2	Condition	Points
C	CHF	1
H	HTN	1
A	75	1
D	DM	1
S$_2$	Prior Stroke/TIA	2

Treatment for CHADS2 Scores	
0 (low risk)	Aspirin
1 (moderate risk)	Aspirin or Oral anticoagulant
2+ (high risk)	Oral anticoagulant

CHADS2 Points	Yearly Stroke Risk (%)
0	1.9
1	2.8
2	4.0
3	5.9
4	8.5
5	12.5
6	18.2

Abbreviations: CHF, congestive heart failure; DM, diabetes mellitus; HTN, hypertension; TIA, transient ischemic attack.

Pulmonary

Many vascular patients have coexisting pulmonary disease, including asthma, emphysema, and chronic obstructive pulmonary disease. Smoking is a risk factor for both vascular and pulmonary disease, and it is not uncommon to find vascular surgery patients who continue to smoke despite their disease. Preoperative pulmonary evaluation tools include chest radiography (CXR), pulmonary function testing (PFTs), and newer testing, such as cardiopulmonary exercise testing.

The focus of preoperative testing should be to identify patients with the highest risk so as to optimize them before elective surgery. Although our primary source of current information about preoperative pulmonary evaluation is from the thoracic surgery patient population, it is difficult to extrapolate these data to the vascular patient population.[25]

Preoperative pulmonary testing should not be used if the result is not going to change intraoperative management or influence overall outcome, as testing is expensive and asymptomatic patients can have abnormal results that do not affect clinical management.[26] Certain patients will benefit from advanced preoperative pulmonary testing, including spirometry or PFTs. This group includes patients with clinical symptoms of cough, dyspnea, or exercise intolerance that cannot be explained by history, physical, or preliminary studies, such as CXR,[27] or those with lung disease undergoing one-lung ventilation for thoracic vascular procedures.

Smoking cessation has been the focus of vascular surgery optimization for decades, primarily because of concerns about wound healing and vascular reocclusion in active smokers.[28] Although some have suggested smoking cessation within 24 hours of surgery may be useful (primarily by reducing carboxyhemoglobin levels), the true clinical benefit of this intervention is likely minimal. Smoking cessation 3 weeks before surgery, however, has been shown to reduce bronchospasm, minimize hypoxemia, reduce cough, and improve tissue oxygenation in the perioperative period.[29]

Finally, many patients with vascular disease suffer from obesity and/or obstructive sleep apnea (OSA). It is estimated that up to 25% of the general patient population has undiagnosed OSA, and identification of this syndrome can be useful in the perioperative care of these patients.[30] All at-risk patients should be screened for OSA by using a tool such as snoring, tired, observed apnea, blood Pressure, body mass index, age, neck circumference, and gender (STOP BANG).[31] Intraoperative considerations for patients with OSA include the recognized difficulty in mask ventilation and intubation, as well as the likelihood for impaired oxygenation and ventilation. Patients with OSA using continuous positive airway pressure devices at home should be instructed to bring the devices with them on the day of surgery for use throughout the perioperative period.[32]

Finally, all patients with preexisting primary or secondary pulmonary disease are at risk for critical postoperative respiratory depression due to residual opioid and anesthetic effects in the setting of compromised respiratory function. A preoperative discussion about the intensity of postoperative observation (eg, intensive care unit, step-down, or ward care) should be routine for this patient population.

Renal

Advances in endovascular surgery have spawned complications not previously seen using open techniques. Many vascular patients, and elderly patients in general, suffer from decreased overall renal function and baseline renal insufficiency is a known risk factor for perioperative morbidity and mortality.[33] This is complicated by the fact that minimally invasive endovascular procedures may require high angiographic dye use to ensure procedural success.

The combination of preexisting renal dysfunction, dye load, and dehydration predisposes these patients to contrast-induced nephropathy (CIN), which is generally defined as a 25% increase in serum creatinine or an absolute increase of 0.5 mg/dL from baseline, following an exposure to contrast.[34] The risk for developing CIN is primarily dependent on baseline renal function, but is also influenced by other risk factors, such as diabetes. The risk for CIN may be less than 2% in patients with normal renal function, even with diabetes. However, in patients with chronic kidney disease, the risk for CIN is inversely proportional to the baseline renal function and is further exacerbated by concurrent diabetes.[35]

Of note, CIN is an even greater concern when inexperienced surgeons or interventionalists perform new procedures, resulting in an increased angiographic dye load. **Boxes 1** and **2** outline patient and contrast-related risk factors, as well as outline preventive strategies to reduce the likelihood or severity of CIN. Identification of patients at risk through appropriate measurement of baseline renal function, along with appropriate preprocedure intravenous hydration, are cornerstones in the prevention of CIN.

Endocrine

Diabetes is a significant risk factor for coronary, cerebral, and peripheral vascular disease, and perioperative glycemic control is an important component of preoperative preparation. Postoperative hyperglycemia results in delayed wound healing, but conversely, attempts at tight glycemic control can result in hypoglycemia and death.[36] Appropriate optimization requires medication management (especially in those taking

Box 1
Patient and nonpatient risk factors for contrast-induced nephropathy

Patient Risk Factors for Contrast-Induced Nephropathy

- Renal disease
- Diabetes mellitus
- Congestive heart failure
- Advanced age
- Anemia
- Left ventricular dysfunction

Nonpatient Risk Factors for Contrast-Induced Nephropathy

- High osmolar contrast load
- Ionic contrast
- Contrast viscosity
- Contrast volume (likely most important and easiest to quantify)

long-acting agents, such as insulin glargine), and appropriate measurement of glucose throughout the perioperative period, with a goal of maintaining serum glucose less than 150 to 160.

Hemoglobin A1c levels also may be a useful preoperative test, as studies of surgical patients have shown a significant incidence of elevated levels in those without a known diagnosis of diabetes[37] and those with elevated hemoglobin A1c may should have appropriate perioperative glucose monitoring. Long-acting oral hypoglycemic agents should be held on the day of surgery. Blood glucose should be measured on presentation to the preoperative area on the day of surgery to help guide the perioperative glucose management plan.

Hematologic

Vascular surgery patients, despite apparent appropriate weight, may suffer from malnutrition and anemia of chronic disease. Anemia, in particular, is independently associated with 30-day death and adverse cardiac events in patients 65 years or older undergoing elective open and endovascular procedures.[38] However, recommendations for laboratory testing must be made on a case-by-case basis depending on age, patient history, medication use, and proposed surgical procedure with its associated risk of blood loss. Not all vascular surgery patients require complete blood count testing before minimally invasive procedures, and not all patients undergoing major procedures require comprehensive blood panels. Guidelines and suggestions

Box 2
Preventative strategies and recommendation to reduce contrast-induced nephropathy

- Check preoperative creatinine in at-risk patients
- In patients at risk, ensure appropriate hydration
- In patients at risk, consider bicarbonate and using low volumes of iso-osmolar or hypo-osmolar contrast solutions
- In patients at high risk, N-acetylcysteine, or ascorbic acid may be beneficial

set forth by the American Society of Anesthesiologists (and others) should be followed based on specific risk.[26]

It is also important to remember that preoperative anticoagulants may have long-lasting effects, necessitating preoperative measurement of prothrombin time (PT) and partial thromboplastin time (PTT). Newer oral anticoagulants do not have a validated preoperative test of anticoagulant effect and one must ensure that patients have ceased the medication for the appropriate period of time before the surgical procedure (see **Table 1**).

Neurologic

Many patients presenting for vascular surgery are elderly with a range of neurologic concerns. These include stroke, transient ischemic attack, dementia and cognitive impairment. Stroke is especially important, as the overall incidence of stroke after noncarotid vascular surgery is 0.6%, with a primary driver being a history of cerebrovascular disease.[39] Prior neurologic conditions may place a patient at great risk for perioperative cognitive decline and confusion, and postoperative delirium that does not fully resolve at time of hospital discharge can result in increased overall morbidity and mortality.[40–42] Specific biomarker analysis, including preoperative serum amyloid-A-protein levels, can be a predictor of poor neurologic outcomes,[43] but indications for these tests are no different in the vascular population than in any other surgical population.

Preexisting neuromuscular deficits in patients with stroke also are a concern. Concurrent arthritic and rheumatoid conditions can amplify weakness in this elderly population. It is therefore important to document baseline strength, mobility, and neurologic deficit in these patients preoperatively, and pay particular attention during positioning at the start of the procedure. Appropriate preoperative optimization, rehabilitation as indicated, and advice about the risks of pain exacerbations are prudent.

One also can tailor the anesthetic approach to improve the recognition of an adverse neurologic condition. For example, multimodal analgesia, including nonopioid analgesics, can reduce postoperative pain and opioid-related side effects; this approach, along with the use of short-acting anesthetics allow for a rapid emergence and neurologic examination while reducing postoperative delirium. When using a regional analgesic technique, it is advisable to minimize the density of the local anesthetic block so that leg weakness due to an intraoperative complication is not masked by local anesthetic–induced numbness and analgesia.

PROCEDURE-SPECIFIC CONSIDERATIONS

Carotid Endarterectomy

Appropriate assessment of the carotid patient requires an understanding of both disease process and proposed surgical technique. Carotid stenosis can be treated via both open and endovascular techniques. Indications for stent placement are complex, and are balanced against a higher incidence of procedural stroke than that seen with open procedures.[44] Although typically performed with sedation anesthesia, appropriate discussion with surgeons and evaluation of patient risk will dictate anesthetic technique and monitoring requirements.

Open carotid endarterectomy may be performed under general anesthesia or with mild sedation and regional block. Advantages of a sedation/regional block technique include the potential for fewer hemodynamic perturbations (eg, during induction and emergence), and the ability for patients to communicate mental status changes during clamping (assuming the sedation is appropriate for this level of communication). Not all patients, however, are candidates for open repair, especially those with morbid obesity, sleep apnea, movement disorders, or claustrophobia.

Aortic Aneurysms

In the era before endovascular surgery, open repair of AAA was challenging, requiring multiple invasive monitors, strict attention to hemodynamics (especially with aortic clamping and unclamping), and anticipation of the likely need for massive transfusion. Newer minimally invasive procedures result in fewer hemodynamic perturbations, and the needs for invasive monitoring and transfusion have therefore lessened.[45] Consequently, patients with more complex comorbidities and or emergent patients now routinely undergo this procedure with minimal morbidity and mortality.[46] Despite this changing landscape, it is still important to understand intraoperative challenges that may be optimized with appropriate preoperative evaluation. One must always keep in mind that a routine endovascular case can rapidly become an open repair, and all of the aforementioned testing guidelines still apply to minimally invasive repairs.

Other preoperative concerns unique to aortic aneurysm surgery include those related to lung isolation and lumbar cerebrospinal fluid drainage. Thoracic aneurysm repair may require thoracotomy, necessitating intubation with lung isolation. Airway evaluation may reveal anatomy that would preclude intubation with a double-lumen tube, and instead favor bronchial blocker placement. Extensive aneurysms may require advanced techniques to prevent spinal cord ischemia, such as lumbar cerebrospinal fluid drainage. History of back surgery, back pain, or intracranial pathology may impact the ability or appropriateness of this procedure.

Lower-Extremity Procedures

Although lower-extremity vascular procedures appear straightforward, patients with peripheral vascular disease still have a high risk of postoperative morbidity and mortality, primarily influenced by concurrent cardiovascular disease in distinction to anesthetic choices.[47] Preoperative testing should focus on comorbidities, risk of CIN, and likelihood of conversion to an open procedure. Many of these patients have had prior vascular surgical procedures, potentially with adverse postoperative complications; a careful history should be obtained to prevent repetition and ameliorate potential postoperative morbidity.

A more unique consideration is that, although many endovascular lower-extremity procedures involve minimal surgical pain, the fluoroscopic tables used can be extremely uncomfortable, making it difficult for older patients or those with chronic back pain to lie still for the duration. Appropriate discussions should be had with patients, and expectations should be addressed as they relate to sedation versus general anesthesia.

Overall Risk Assessment

Risk identification and reduction are significant elements to the preoperative assessment. Traditionally, morbidity and mortality after surgical procedures are attributable to (1) baseline comorbid conditions, (2) the surgical procedure itself, and (3) the anesthetic management.[40] Risk stratification primarily depends on the type and control of a comorbid condition, along with the impact of the procedure on the patient. Specific risk categories are cardiac and pulmonary conditions, as complications in these 2 organ systems drive long-term mortality after vascular surgery.[48]

Others have noted the importance of urgent surgery, baseline creatinine greater than 3.5 mg/dL, congestive heart failure, and ventricular arrhythmias to identify poor long-term outcomes after vascular surgery.[33] Specific surgical concerns also enter into a risk assessment, such as aortic diameter for thoracic endovascular surgery[49] and the high risk of mortality after amputation.[50] Many have created risk scores to predict perioperative morbidity and mortality and 2 example scores are the older RCRI (Revised Cardiac Risk Index) for stratification of patients undergoing noncardiac surgery[51] and the NSQIP (National Surgical Quality Improvement Project) score.[52] Of note, some have questioned the validity of the RCRI in vascular surgical patients, although it is a popular tool.[53] The NSQIP risk calculator has been turned into an online tool for easy use during preoperative assessment.[54]

SUMMARY AND FUTURE CONSIDERATIONS

Patients requiring vascular surgery present a multitude of perioperative challenges despite a recent move toward less-invasive procedures. These patients frequently suffer from a host of significant comorbidities that must be identified and addressed before surgical and anesthetic care. As endovascular procedures continue to evolve, our anesthetic preoperative evaluation and planning also must evolve. The core principles of excellent patient assessment and preparation will need to be continually evaluated in the context of changing surgical need. As always, lifelong learning and close communication with our surgical colleagues will ensure that we provide the safest care possible to our patients while reducing risk and optimizing patient outcomes.

REFERENCES

1. Feringa HH, Karagiannis SE, Vidakovic R, et al. The prevalence and prognosis of unrecognized myocardial infarction and silent myocardial ischemia in patients undergoing major vascular surgery. Coron Artery Dis 2007;18(7):571–6.
2. Schwarze ML, Shen Y, Hemmerich J, et al. Age-related trends in utilization and outcome of open and endovascular repair for abdominal aortic aneurysm in the United States, 2001-2006. J Vasc Surg 2009;50(4):722–9.e2.
3. Fleisher LA, Beckman JA, Brown KA, et al. ACC/AHA 2007 guidelines on perioperative cardiovascular evaluation and care for noncardiac surgery: executive summary: a report of the American College of Cardiology/American Heart Association task force on practice guidelines (Writing Committee to revise the 2002 guidelines on perioperative cardiovascular evaluation for noncardiac surgery) developed in Collaboration With the American Society of Echocardiography, American Society of Nuclear Cardiology, Heart Rhythm Society, Society of Cardiovascular Anesthesiologists, Society for Cardiovascular Angiography and Interventions, Society for Vascular Medicine and Biology, and Society for Vascular Surgery. J Am Coll Cardiol 2007;50(17):1707–32.
4. Grines CL, Bonow RO, Casey DE, et al. Prevention of premature discontinuation of dual antiplatelet therapy in patients with coronary artery stents: a science advisory from the American Heart Association, American College of Cardiology, Society for Cardiovascular Angiography and Interventions, American College of Surgeons, and American Dental Association, with representation from the American College of Physicians. J Am Coll Cardiol 2007;49(6):734–9.
5. Hawn MT, Graham LA, Richman JS, et al. Risk of major adverse cardiac events following noncardiac surgery in patients with coronary stents. JAMA 2013;310(14):1462–72.
6. Clerico A, Emdin M, Passino C. Cardiac biomarkers and risk assessment in patients undergoing major non-cardiac surgery: time to revise the guidelines? Clin Chem Lab Med 2014;52:959–63.

7. Causey MW, Mcvay DP, Oguntoye M, et al. Application of preoperative brain natriuretic peptide levels in clinical practice. Vascular 2013;21(4):225–31.
8. Biccard BM, Naidoo P, De vasconcellos K. What is the best pre-operative risk stratification tool for major adverse cardiac events following elective vascular surgery? A prospective observational cohort study evaluating pre-operative myocardial ischaemia monitoring and biomarker analysis. Anaesthesia 2012; 67(4):389–95.
9. Fleisher LA, Beckman JA, Brown KA, et al. 2009 ACCF/AHA focused update on perioperative beta blockade incorporated into the ACC/AHA 2007 guidelines on perioperative cardiovascular evaluation and care for noncardiac surgery. J Am Coll Cardiol 2009;54(22):e13–118.
10. White CM, Talati R, Phung OJ, et al. Benefits and risks associated with beta-blocker prophylaxis in noncardiac surgery. Am J Health Syst Pharm 2010; 67(7):523–30.
11. Devereaux PJ, Yang H, Yusuf S, et al. Effects of extended-release metoprolol succinate in patients undergoing non-cardiac surgery (POISE trial): a randomized controlled trial. Lancet 2008;371(9627):1839–47.
12. Foex P, Sear JW. II. β-Blockers and cardiac protection: 5 yr on from POISE. Br J Anaesth 2014;112(2):206–10.
13. Heidbuchel H, Verhamme P, Alings M, et al. EHRA practical guide on the use of new oral anticoagulants in patients with non-valvular atrial fibrillation: executive summary. Eur Heart J 2013;34(27):2094–106.
14. Spyropoulos AC, Douketis JD. How I treat anticoagulated patients undergoing an elective procedure or surgery. Blood 2012;120(15):2954–62.
15. Nitzki-george D, Wozniak I, Caprini JA. Current state of knowledge on oral anticoagulant reversal using procoagulant factors. Ann Pharmacother 2013;47(6):841–55.
16. Harrison RW, Ortel TL, Becker RC. To bridge or not to bridge: these are the questions. J Thromb Thrombolysis 2012;34(1):31–5.
17. Benzon HT, Avram MJ, Green D, et al. New oral anticoagulants and regional anaesthesia. Br J Anaesth 2013;111(Suppl 1):i96–113.
18. Schouten O, Boersma E, Hoeks SE, et al. Fluvastatin and perioperative events in patients undergoing vascular surgery. N Engl J Med 2009;361(10):980–9.
19. Feldman LS, Brotman DJ. Perioperative statins: more than lipid-lowering? Cleve Clin J Med 2008;75(9):654–62.
20. Le Manach Y, Ibanez Esteves C, Bertrand M, et al. Impact of preoperative statin therapy on adverse postoperative outcomes in patients undergoing vascular surgery. Anesthesiology 2011;114(1):98–104.
21. Moulakakis KG, Matoussevitch V, Borgonio A, et al. Evidence that statins protect renal function during endovascular repair of AAAs. Eur J Vasc Endovasc Surg 2010;40(5):608–15.
22. Paraskevas KI, Mikhailidis DP, Veith FJ. Optimal statin type and dosage for vascular patients. J Vasc Surg 2011;53(3):837–44.
23. Durazzo AE, Machado FS, Ikeoka DT, et al. Reduction in cardiovascular events after vascular surgery with atorvastatin: a randomized trial. J Vasc Surg 2004; 39(5):967–75.
24. Paraskevas KI, Veith FJ, Liapis CD, et al. Perioperative/periprocedural effects of statin treatment for patients undergoing vascular surgery or endovascular procedures: an update. Curr Vasc Pharmacol 2013;11(1):112–20.
25. Young EL, Karthikesalingam A, Huddart S, et al. A systematic review of the role of cardiopulmonary exercise testing in vascular surgery. Eur J Vasc Endovasc Surg 2012;44(1):64–71.

26. Apfelbaum JL, Connis RT, Nickinovich DG, et al. Practice advisory for preanesthesia evaluation: an updated report by the American Society of Anesthesiologists task force on preanesthesia evaluation. Anesthesiology 2012;116(3): 522–38.
27. Bernstein WK. Pulmonary function testing. Curr Opin Anaesthesiol 2012;25(1): 11–6.
28. Kraiss LW, Johansen K. Pharmacologic intervention to prevent graft failure. Surg Clin North Am 1995;75(4):761–72.
29. Wong J, Lam DP, Abrishami A, et al. Short-term preoperative smoking cessation and postoperative complications: a systematic review and meta-analysis. Can J Anaesth 2012;59(3):268–79.
30. Young T, Peppard PE, Gottlieb DJ. Epidemiology of obstructive sleep apnea: a population health perspective. Am J Respir Crit Care Med 2002;165(9): 1217–39.
31. Seet E, Chung F. Obstructive sleep apnea: preoperative assessment. Anesthesiol Clin 2010;28(2):199–215.
32. Gross JB, Bachenberg KL, Benumof JL, et al. Practice guidelines for the perioperative management of patients with obstructive sleep apnea: a report by the American Society of Anesthesiologists task force on perioperative management of patients with obstructive sleep apnea. Anesthesiology 2006;104(5): 1081–93.
33. Mcfalls EO, Ward HB, Moritz TE, et al. Clinical factors associated with long-term mortality following vascular surgery: outcomes from the Coronary Artery Revascularization Prophylaxis (CARP) Trial. J Vasc Surg 2007;46(4):694–700.
34. Barrett B, Parfrey P. Preventing nephropathy induced by contrast medium. N Engl J Med 2006;354:379–86.
35. Rudnick M, Goldfarb S, Tumlin J. Contrast-induced nephropathy: is the picture any clearer? Clin J Am Soc Nephrol 2008;3:261–2.
36. Lipshutz AK, Gropper MA. Perioperative glycemic control: an evidence-based review. Anesthesiology 2009;110(2):408–21.
37. Wexler DJ, Nathan DM, Grant RW, et al. Prevalence of elevated hemoglobin A1c among patients admitted to the hospital without a diagnosis of diabetes. J Clin Endocrinol Metab 2008;93(11):4238–44.
38. Gupta PK, Sundaram A, Mactaggart JN, et al. Preoperative anemia is an independent predictor of postoperative mortality and adverse cardiac events in elderly patients undergoing elective vascular operations. Ann Surg 2013; 258(6):1096–102.
39. Sharifpour M, Moore LE, Shanks AM, et al. Incidence, predictors, and outcomes of perioperative stroke in noncarotid major vascular surgery. Anesth Analg 2013; 116(2):424–34.
40. Monk TG, Saini V, Weldon BC, et al. Anesthetic management and one-year mortality after noncardiac surgery. Anesth Analg 2005;100(1):4–10.
41. Price CC, Garvan CW, Monk TG. Type and severity of cognitive decline in older adults after noncardiac surgery. Anesthesiology 2008;108(1):8–17.
42. Deiner S, Silverstein JH. Postoperative delirium and cognitive dysfunction. Br J Anaesth 2009;103(Suppl 1):i41–6.
43. Pini R, Faggioli G, Fittipaldi S, et al. Inflammatory mediators and cerebral embolism in carotid stenting: new markers of risk. J Endovasc Ther 2013;20(5): 684–94.
44. Touzé E, Trinquart L, Felgueiras R, et al. A clinical rule (sex, contralateral occlusion, age, and restenosis) to select patients for stenting versus carotid

endarterectomy: systematic review of observational studies with validation in randomized trials. Stroke 2013;44(12):3394–400.
45. Subramaniam K, Park KW, Subramaniam B. Anesthesia and perioperative care for the vascular patient. Br J Anaesth 2013;111(4):682–3.
46. Hogendoorn W, Schlösser F, Muhs B, et al. Surgical and anesthetic considerations for the endovascular treatment of ruptured descending thoracic aortic aneurysms. Curr Opin Anaesthesiol 2014;27(1):12–20.
47. Ghanami RJ, Hurie J, Andrews JS, et al. Anesthesia-based evaluation of outcomes of lower-extremity vascular bypass procedures. Ann Vasc Surg 2013;27(2):199–207.
48. Orcutt ST, Bechara CF, Pisimisis G, et al. Impact of perioperative events on mortality after major vascular surgery in a veteran patient population. Am J Surg 2012;204(5):586–90.
49. Shah AA, Craig DM, Andersen ND, et al. Risk factors for 1-year mortality after thoracic endovascular aortic repair. J Thorac Cardiovasc Surg 2013;145(5):1242–7.
50. Jones WS, Patel MR, Dai D, et al. High mortality risks after major lower extremity amputation in Medicare patients with peripheral artery disease. Am Heart J 2013;165(5):809–15, 815.e1.
51. Lee TH, Marcantonio ER, Mangione CM, et al. Derivation and prospective validation of a simple index for prediction of cardiac risk of major noncardiac surgery. Circulation 1999;100(10):1043–9.
52. Bilimoria KY, Liu Y, Paruch JL, et al. Development and evaluation of the universal ACS NSQIP surgical risk calculator: a decision aid and informed consent tool for patients and surgeons. J Am Coll Surg 2013;217(5):833–42.e1–3.
53. Payne CJ, Bryce GJ, Gibson SC, et al. The revised cardiac risk index performs poorly in patients undergoing major vascular surgery: a prospective observational study. Eur J Anaesthesiol 2013;30(11):713–5.
54. NSQIP on-line risk calculator. Available at: http://riskcalculator.facs.org/. Accessed February 27, 2013.

Optimal Perioperative Medical Management of the Vascular Surgery Patient

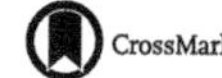

Saket Singh, MD*, Yasdet Maldonado, MD, Mark A. Taylor, MD

KEYWORDS

• Vascular surgery • Carotid stenosis • Abdominal aortic aneurysm • Troponin leak • β-blocker • Glucose control • Anesthesia • Cerebral hyperperfusion

KEY POINTS

- Moderate tight glucose control is currently the safest approach for patients undergoing vascular surgery.
- Use of statins during the perioperative period decreases complications during vascular surgery.
- General anesthesia should be avoided, when possible, for endovascular abdominal aortic aneurysm repair.
- Risk stratification based on troponin leak can be considered for patients undergoing vascular surgery.
- In patients undergoing carotid artery endarterectomies cerebral near-infrared spectroscopy can help detect cerebral hyperperfusion, which can be prevented with early identification and control of blood pressure.

INTRODUCTION

High-risk vascular patients undergoing complicated procedures can benefit from anesthesia providers managing preoperative, intraoperative, and postoperative care. As health care evolves, comprehensive perioperative management of patients will become more dependent on involvement of anesthesiologists in the delivery of high-quality, evidence-based medicine to all surgical patients.

PREOPERATIVE MANAGEMENT

Preoperative management of patients undergoing vascular surgery can be complicated because these patients often have coexisting cardiac, pulmonary, cerebrovascular,

Disclosure: The authors have no conflicts of interest.

Department of Anesthesiology, Allegheny Health Network, Temple University School of Medicine, 2570 Haymaker Road, Pittsburgh, PA 15146, USA
* Corresponding author.
E-mail address: ssingh@wpahs.org

Anesthesiology Clin 32 (2014) 615–637
http://dx.doi.org/10.1016/j.anclin.2014.05.007 **anesthesiology.theclinics.com**
1932-2275/14/$ – see front matter

endocrine, and renal comorbidities. A preoperative evaluation should focus on optimizing comorbid conditions and minimizing perioperative risk.

Cardiovascular Evaluation

Major vascular surgeries represent the highest-risk procedures for cardiovascular morbidity and mortality.[1] Open vascular surgery, such as repairs of the aorta and visceral arteries, and lower limb revascularization, is considered high risk, whereas endovascular repairs, carotid endarterectomies, and percutaneous extremity angioplasties should be considered intermediate risk.[1,2] Dialysis access procedures, varicose vein procedures, and minor amputations involving digits should be considered low risk.[2] Any emergent or urgent vascular surgery should be considered high risk.[2]

As the prevalence of coronary artery disease (CAD) is approximately 50% in patients undergoing vascular surgery,[3] a 12 lead electrocardiogram should be considered for all patients presenting for surgery. Stress testing is not predictive of myocardial morbidity or mortality, and should only be recommended in patients with unstable angina or an active arrhythmia.[4,5] In these patients, exercise stress testing should be performed when possible. In patients unable to exercise, which is not uncommon in vascular surgery patients, dobutamine stress echocardiography (DSE) or myocardial perfusion scintigraphy can help predict perioperative cardiac events in patients undergoing noncardiac surgery. If there are signs of active ischemia and the patient is symptomatic, he or she should undergo coronary angiography.[4]

Analysis of the results of the Coronary Artery Revascularization Prophylaxis (CARP) trial reveals that the only groups who benefit from revascularization before vascular surgery are those with unstable CAD or left main coronary artery disease.[2,6,7] For patients proceeding with surgery, percutaneous coronary intervention (PCI) can proceed preferably 6 weeks after surgery.[2] After successful PCI, vascular surgery should ideally be scheduled at least 1 month after deployment of a bare-metal stent and 1 year after drug-eluting stent deployment, to decrease the risk of stent thrombosis secondary to discontinuing dual-antiplatelet therapy prematurely.

A large, multicenter, prospective review by Stone and colleagues[8] demonstrated that clopidogrel is not associated with major bleeding complications after vascular surgery. In this study, patients in whom clopidogrel was continued either alone or as part of dual-antiplatelet therapy did not have significant bleeding complications, including reoperation or transfusion, compared with patients on aspirin alone or no therapy. Saadeh and Sfeir[9] confirmed these findings in a prospective, nonrandomized study demonstrating that dual-antiplatelet therapy up to the day of surgery is also not associated with bleeding complications. Hence, clopidogrel and/or dual-antiplatelet therapy may be safely continued in patients with recent stents or those with symptomatic carotid disease when surgery is necessary before completion of the recommended course of therapy.

There is debate regarding the optimal timing for elective vascular surgery following revascularization via coronary artery bypass grafting (CABG). A retrospective review by Paty and colleagues[10] concluded that repair of large abdominal aortic aneurysms (AAAs) should be performed early (median interprocedure interval of 11.5 days) after CABG to decrease the interprocedural risk of rupture. Hence, the timing of vascular surgery after CABG needs to be determined on an individual basis, taking into account the urgency of the vascular surgery, the risks of rupture or worsening vascular disease in the immediate postoperative cardiac surgery period, and the risks of early and late cardiac events.

In patients presenting for emergent or urgent surgery with a questionable cardiac history, the anesthesiologist with expertise in perioperative echocardiography may perform a focused transthoracic echocardiogram (FoCUS).[11] Indications for FoCUS examination include, but are not limited to, hemodynamic instability, undifferentiated murmur/valve disease, assessment of ventricular function, dyspnea/hypoxemia, and poor functional capacity.[12] The specific views for the FoCUS examination are at the discretion of the anesthesiologist but may include those listed in **Box 1**. Findings typically correlate 90% of the time with those of a formal examination, and help to tailor perioperative management.[12]

β-Blockers

The use of β-blockers within the perioperative period has been strongly debated over the past decade. All patients undergoing vascular surgery, except those without risk factors, should be considered for β-blocker therapy.[4] According to the most recent update in 2009 from the American College of Cardiology/American Heart Association (ACC/AHA), β-blockers should be continued perioperatively in those patients already taking them preoperatively (Class I recommendation).[13] Withdrawal of β-blockers postoperatively in this patient population undergoing vascular surgery will lead to an increase in cardiovascular morbidity and mortality.[14] In addition, those patients undergoing high-risk vascular surgery who also have major comorbidities including inducible ischemia, CAD, or other multiple clinical risk factors should receive β-blockade (Class IIa recommendation).[13]

The POISE trial elucidated the complications that may occur following the initiation of high-dose β-blockade on the day of surgery.[15] Prophylactic β-blockers may be useful to reduce the incidence of myocardial ischemia but are also associated with an increased risk of bradycardia and hypotension (**Table 1**).[16] If administered, β-blockade should be titrated at an appropriate preoperative interval, typically 7 days, but preferably 30 days, before surgery, to adjust for bradycardia, hypotension, and so forth,[13,17,18] and should be titrated with a goal heart rate of 60 to 80 beats per minute.[13] The American College of Cardiology Foundation/American Heart Association (ACCF/AHA) recommends to hold β-blockade if the patient experiences hypotension (exact pressure undefined).[13]

Controversy also still exists regarding the best β-blocker formulation to use for perioperative patients. A large observational study by Wallace and colleagues[19]

Box 1
Checklist of recommended items to include in a focused transthoracic echocardiography examination

- Right ventricle size and function (2D)
- Left ventricle size and function (2D)
- Ejection fraction (2D)
- Tricuspid valve, including right ventricular systolic pressure (2D, CFD, CWD)
- Mitral valve (2D, CFD)
- Aortic valve, including velocity/gradient (2D, CFD, CWD)
- IVC and collapsibility (2D)

Abbreviations: 2D, 2-dimensional imaging; CFD, color-flow Doppler; CWD, continuous-wave Doppler; IVC, inferior vena cava.

Data from Cowie B. Three years experience of focused cardiovascular ultrasound in the perioperative period. Anaesthesia 2011;66(4):268–73.

Table 1
Effect of perioperative β-blockade therapy

Outcome	Noncardiac Surgery	Cardiac Surgery
All-cause mortality	No effect	No effect
Myocardial infarction	No effect	No effect
Myocardial ischemia	Reduced	No effect
Ventricular arrhythmias	No effect	Reduced
Atrial fibrillation/flutter Supraventricular arrhythmias	No effect	Reduced
Length of hospitalization	No effect	No effect
Perioperative bradycardia	Increased	Increased
Hypotension	Increased	Increased

Data from Wiesbauer F, Schlager O, Domanovits H, et al. Perioperative beta-blockers for preventing surgery-related mortality and morbidity: a systematic review and meta-analysis. Anesth Analg 2007;104(1):37.

demonstrated that atenolol decreased mortality at both 30 days and 1 year when compared with metoprolol. Preoperative metoprolol, but not atenolol, is also associated with stroke after noncardiac surgery.[20] The risk of stroke with metoprolol, but not esmolol or labetalol, extends into the intraoperative period.[20] Bisoprolol is also being evaluated as an alternative agent to metoprolol.[21] In patients on chronic β-blocker therapy, the same β-blocker class should be continued perioperatively.[2] Owing to potential research misconduct in several of the trials that have formed the foundation for the perioperative β-blockade literature, further randomized clinical trials need to be undertaken to better define best practice for perioperative β-blockade.

Treatment of Hypertension

β-Blockers, α-blockers, and angiotensin-converting enzyme (ACE) inhibitors are common antihypertensive agents found on the medication lists of patients scheduled for vascular surgery. In a retrospective study by Hirsch and colleagues,[22] β-blockers were shown to potentially decrease the risk of AAA rupture. By contrast, an association was recently found between chronic renin-angiotensin system (RAS) blockade and increased 30-day mortality after AAA repair.[23] Debate continues regarding the perioperative cessation of these medications and its impact on postoperative outcomes.

There is also discussion as to the possible relationship between RAS-blocking drugs and anesthetic agents.[23] Inhaled anesthetics inhibit protein kinase C, an enzyme involved in signaling pathways, leading to decreased activity of the angiotensin-1 receptor and increased activity of the angiotensin-2 receptor, ultimately culminating in decreased vascular tone.[23] As a result, hypertensive agents such as β-blockers and α-blockers should be continued on the day of surgery, but consideration should be given on an individual basis to holding ACE inhibitors, angiotensin II receptor blockers, and diuretics.

Statins

Vascular surgery patients on statin therapy preoperatively should receive statins in the perioperative period, and their use is reasonable in such patients, both with and without clinical risk factors, who are not on statin therapy preoperatively.[24] Statins have been demonstrated to provide a protective effect against cardiac complications for noncardiac surgery, and their use during the perioperative period can potentially decrease complications following vascular surgery.[24]

Smoking Cessation

Smoking cessation reduces cardiovascular, respiratory, and wound-related complications. Observational studies have demonstrated that amputation, myocardial infarction, and risk of death are higher in smokers.[25] Likewise, lower extremity angioplasty patency rates are also lower in this patient population.[25] Nicotine has a short half-life of 1 to 2 hours, so even a brief reprieve from smoking has benefits, although long-term cessation is optimal.

A study by Woehlck and colleagues[26] in vascular surgery patients without ischemic heart disease demonstrated that patients who continued smoking until the morning of surgery had higher incidences of ST-segment depression compared with both nonsmokers and smokers who did not smoke before surgery. Historically, studies were published suggesting that quitting smoking on the day of surgery would increase the risk of complications; however, more recent studies do not support these conclusions.[27] It is especially important that patients with thromboangiitis obliterans be counseled to stop smoking, as smoking is thought to be a primary causative factor in this syndrome.[25]

Smoking also increases the risk of stroke by 25% to 50%.[28] This fact is particularly important in patients suffering from carotid stenosis, as smoking enhances progression of the stenosis. Prospective randomized trials need to be undertaken to determine the effects of smoking cessation on morbidity and mortality of patients undergoing vascular surgery. The American Society of Anesthesiologists has a Web site titled "Be Smoke Free for Surgery" that provides tools for the anesthesiologist to help patients quit smoking (www.asahq.org/stopsmoking).

Antiplatelet Drugs

Aspirin and clopidogrel have both been used successfully to reduce the risk of myocardial infarction, stroke, and death.[25] Dual-antiplatelet therapy with aspirin and clopidogrel is essential in reducing cardiac risk after coronary stent implantation. As previously stated, elective procedures should be deferred until at least 1 month after placement of a bare-metal stent and 12 months after placement of a drug-eluting stent in order for the patient to receive appropriate therapy.[29]

If surgery is necessary before the recommended wait period, consideration should be given to at least continuing aspirin therapy and restarting clopidogrel as soon as possible postoperatively or continuing dual therapy perioperatively.[8,9] Consideration should also be given to continuing aspirin after the 12-month period for drug-eluting stents to decrease the risk of in-stent thrombosis.[30]

In patients who have suffered a previous ischemic stroke, either monotherapy (aspirin, clopidogrel) or combination therapy such as aspirin plus dipyridamole is recommended.[28,31] Aspirin does not create a level of risk if regional anesthesia is going to be performed, but clopidogrel should be discontinued 7 days before a neuraxial block.[32] There is a lack of data regarding regional anesthetics and dipyridamole, but current guidelines suggest that when used alone there is no need for discontinuation before neuraxial blockade.[32]

Herbal medications may also provide an antiplatelet effect, specifically the 3 Gs: garlic, gingko, and ginseng. Garlic is known to irreversibly inhibit platelet aggregation and may potentiate the effect of other antiplatelet drugs.[33] Garlic should be stopped 7 days before surgery.[32,34] Gingko may also inhibit and alter platelet function, and should be stopped at least 36 hours before surgery.[32–34] Ginseng inhibits platelet aggregation and should be stopped 24 hours before surgery.[32] Continuing herbal medications alone up to the day of surgery is not a contraindication for regional anesthesia, but the American Society of Regional Anesthesia warns that if the patient is on a prescribed antiplatelet agent and is also taking a herbal medication, the practitioner should proceed with caution, as the specific combined effect is unknown.[32]

Diabetes Mellitus

Diabetes mellitus confers a 2-fold risk for CAD, stroke, and death.[35] There is also a moderate association in diabetics between the specific impaired fasting glucose level with coronary artery disease and stroke.[35] Diabetes has been identified as a clinical risk factor by the ACC and AHA, and further preoperative cardiac evaluation is recommended in diabetic patients undergoing vascular surgery who have poor functional status or additional risk factors.[1]

Diabetes and hyperglycemia lead to an impairment of nitric oxide function.[36] Nitric oxide is the major contributor to endothelium relaxation in arteries. In addition, both type 1 and type 2 diabetics have decreased levels of endothelial progenitor cells (EPCs).[36] Endothelial repair is mediated through EPCs,[36] and there is a direct relationship between hyperglycemia and impaired proliferation, survival, and function of EPCs. Insulin therapy can restore EPC function to normal.[36]

Diabetic patients undergoing vascular surgery should ideally be optimized to the extent of having a goal hemoglobin A1c of less than 7%.[37] Oral hypoglycemic agents should be discontinued the day before surgery, with the exception of chlorpropamide, which should be stopped 2 days before surgery. A large retrospective review by McGirt and colleagues[38] evaluated the association between hyperglycemia and stroke, myocardial infarction, and death in patients undergoing the most common noncardiac vascular procedure, carotid endarterectomy.

Moderately tight glucose control is currently the safest approach for patients undergoing vascular surgery. Patients with a preoperative glucose greater than 200 mg/dL were 4.3-fold, 2.8-fold, and 3.3-fold more likely to experience a myocardial infarction, perioperative stroke or transient ischemic attack, or death, respectively. Based on a review of randomized controlled trials and meta-analyses by Van Kuijk and colleagues,[39] a target glucose level of 108 to 150 mg/dL appears to be beneficial. However, insulin protocols are rarely begun preoperatively, largely because of the fear of hypoglycemia, and many diabetics with vascular disease are on β-blockers, medications that can mask the symptoms of hypoglycemia by blocking the effects of the catecholamine release induced by hypoglycemia.[40] Nevertheless, the anesthesiologist should use clinical judgment and institutional protocols when deciding to treat hyperglycemia perioperatively.

Renal

Patients with vascular disease may have concomitant renal disease resulting from hypertensive nephropathy, diabetic nephropathy, or renal artery stenosis.[41] These patients should have a preoperative complete blood count to evaluate for anemia and thrombocytopenia, and should also be evaluated for electrolyte and acid-base abnormalities. Baseline renal function should be determined, as renal insufficiency is a clinical risk factor for cardiovascular complications. Dialysis patients (end-stage renal disease) should have dialysis performed on the day before surgery to decrease the risk of volume overload, hyperkalemia, and bleeding from uremia.

INTRAOPERATIVE MANAGEMENT

Most patients undergoing vascular surgery are at high risk secondary to multiple comorbidities. These patients are very challenging because most vascular surgical procedures induce tremendous oxygen demand and supply imbalance caused by arterial cross-clamping, acute changes in blood pressure, ischemia, and sudden metabolic changes, leading to higher perioperative morbidity and mortality.

Monitoring

All vascular procedures requiring anesthesia should be monitored with standard American Society of Anesthesiology (ASA) monitors. The use of advanced monitors, such as an arterial line, central venous catheter, pulmonary artery catheter, transesophageal echocardiogram, and minimally invasive continuous cardiac output monitor, will depend on patient risk factors, type of procedure and anesthetic, availability of equipment, and, most importantly, the anesthesiologist's expertise and preference.

A recent prospective, randomized, multicenter study by Scheeren and colleagues[42] demonstrated that patients undergoing procedures involving large fluid shifts may benefit from intravascular volume administration based on stroke-volume variation and pulse-pressure variation. Goal-directed intraoperative fluid therapy has been shown to decrease the incidence of postoperative wound infections, and may have decreased postoperative organ dysfunction. Romagnoli and colleagues[43] conducted a prospective observational study that compared the FloTrac/Vigileo cardiac output (Edwards Lifesciences, Irvine, CA, USA) and the MostCare/PRAM cardiac output (Vytec Health, Padova, Italy) with transthoracic echocardiographic cardiac output estimations (reference method). In patients undergoing vascular surgery, the FloTrac/Vigileo did not demonstrate that it was a reliable system for cardiac output monitoring when compared with echocardiography-derived cardiac output. However, MostCare/PRAM was shown to estimate cardiac output with a good level of agreement with echocardiographic measures.

Fluid Management

Optimal fluid management of patients undergoing major vascular surgery has been the subject of much debate and controversy for many years, especially in those with AAAs. The most recent trials describe an improvement in outcomes with a restrictive fluid management strategy. Positive fluid balances, prolonged operative and cross-clamp times, and large blood loss are independent predictors of complications such as cardiopulmonary dysfunction and acute renal failure.[44]

The Cochrane Peripheral Vascular Diseases Group reviewed data from 38 randomized controlled trials and found that fluid type (crystalloid vs colloid) does not affect any outcome measure.[45] Bunn and Trivedi[46] analyzed randomized controlled trials in critically ill and surgical patients, and did not find any evidence that one colloid solution is more effective or safe than another. The current evidence suggests that all hydroxyethyl starch products increase the risk of acute kidney injury requiring renal replacement therapy in all patient populations.[47] Because the optimal safe volume for hydroxyethyl starch has not been determined, the risks outweigh the benefits; therefore, alternative volume replacement therapies should be used.

Anemia

Perioperative blood transfusion guidelines published by the ASA should be referenced for the vascular surgery patient, with special consideration given to the patient on β-blockers. An observational study by Le Manach and colleagues[48] involving patients receiving chronic β-blockade and undergoing infrarenal aortic reconstructive surgery demonstrated that severe bleeding was more common in β-blocked patients. Hence, higher transfusion thresholds may be necessary in the β-blocked patient undergoing major vascular surgery.[21]

Carotid Endarterectomies

At present there are 3 different anesthetic options available for carotid endarterectomies: general (GA), regional (RA), or a combination of both. Schechter and colleagues[49] used the American College of Surgeons National Surgical Quality Improvement Program (NSQIP) to evaluate the influence of anesthesia modality on outcomes after carotid endarterectomy. There was no difference in the rate of complications for the entire study population of 24,716 patients and the propensity-matched cohort of 8050 patients. **Box 2** lists the most common complications associated with carotid endarterectomies. The General Anesthesia versus Local Anesthesia (GALA) trial, which represents the only large, multicenter, randomized controlled trial comparing GA with RA for carotid endarterectomies, found no difference in postoperative outcomes between anesthesia modalities.[50]

General anesthesia is still the most frequently performed modality for carotid endarterectomies.[51,52] The advantages of a GA include the following: secure airway, potential benefits of ischemic preconditioning, neuroprotection conferred by the use of inhalational agents and/or propofol, possible greater surgeon satisfaction, and possible greater patient satisfaction.

Patients under GA may tolerate lower stump pressures attributable to the potential protective effect of the inhalational agents, which decrease the cerebral metabolic rate for oxygen. However, some studies indicate that higher rates of shunting are observed in patients receiving GA (20%–30%) when compared with patients receiving RA with cervical plexus blocks (5%–10%).[53] In addition, GA is associated with longer operative times and is more likely to result in patients remaining hospitalized beyond the first postoperative day.[54]

Some surgeons favor regional anesthesia (superficial and/or deep cervical plexus block) because they believe an awake patient is the most reliable monitor for detecting cerebral ischemia. RA also avoids the deleterious hemodynamic and pulmonary

Box 2
Complications associated with carotid revascularization

- Stroke or transient ischemic attack
- Myocardial ischemia or Infarction
- Wound hematoma
- Cranial nerve injury
- Intracerebral hemorrhage
- Seizures
- Hypertension
- Hypotension
- Bradycardia
- Airway obstruction
- Arrhythmias

complications associated with general anesthesia and airway instrumentation. However, other complications may arise including, but not limited to, the following: risk for a failed block (2%),[55] hemidiaphragmatic paralysis, inadvertent total spinal block, and seizure. In addition, once the procedure is under way there is limited access to the patient with an unsecured airway; patient-anxiety issues may also arise. Some of the complications associated with a deep cervical plexus blocks can be avoided or reduced by performing only a superficial cervical plexus block or by performing the block under ultrasound guidance.

The third anesthetic option is a combined regional and general anesthetic. In this technique, a superficial cervical plexus block is performed, followed by induction of GA. The patient is placed on a high-dose remifentanil infusion, which is stopped at the time of clamping so that the patient is awake and collaborating within a few minutes. During the course of 6 years, Marcucci and colleagues[56] prospectively evaluated the usefulness of a combined anesthetic, and found that the GA component provided hemodynamic stability and excellent control of ventilation while the RA component provided ease of evaluation of neurologic status in a calm and relaxed environment for both the patient and surgeon.

The ideal anesthetic technique for carotid endarterectomies remains a matter of debate. The analysis from pooled data from randomized controlled trials shows that there is no clear evidence in favor of one anesthetic technique over another, and the choice should be based on the clinical situation, along with the preference of the patient and medical providers involved.

Abdominal Aortic Aneurysms

Open abdominal aortic aneurysms

Open abdominal aortic aneurysm repairs can be performed under general anesthesia, neuraxial anesthesia, or a combination of both. Current literature does not clearly show long-term benefit of one form of anesthesia over another. Nishimori and colleagues[57] analyzed data from all randomized and quasi-randomized controlled trials from the inception of the Cochrane database until 2010 that compared postoperative epidural analgesia and systemic opioid-based analgesia for adult patients who underwent elective open abdominal aortic surgery. Epidural analgesia was found to provide better pain relief during the first 3 postoperative days. It also reduced the duration of postoperative tracheal intubation by roughly 50%. The occurrence of prolonged postoperative mechanical ventilation, myocardial infarction, gastric complications, and renal complications were also reduced by epidural analgesia. However, the investigators concluded that current evidence does not confirm the beneficial effect of epidural analgesia in preventing postoperative mortality.

A recent prospective cohort study by Licker and colleagues[58] also evaluated the impact of anesthetic technique on the incidence of major complications after open abdominal aortic surgery. Patients who received thoracic epidural analgesia required routine vasopressor use to maintain stable hemodynamics. The intraoperative use of vasopressors is an independent risk factor for acute kidney injury.[59] Patients managed with thoracic epidural analgesia or given intrathecal morphine required lower doses of intravenous analgesia intraoperatively and were extubated sooner than those who received systemic analgesia.

Intrathecal morphine was also associated with a lower risk of postoperative morbidity, specifically pulmonary and renal complications. In addition, a more restrictive fluid regimen was achieved in the patients who received intrathecal morphine when compared with the group that received systemic analgesia, which required larger fluid volumes (on average approximately 2400 mL greater). These results suggest that the administration of intrathecal morphine as part of a combined anesthetic may reduce the rate of perioperative complications in major vascular surgery.

Finally, transverse abdominis plane (TAP) blocks have been demonstrated to be effective pain relief adjuncts in upper abdominal surgeries.[60] Bilateral TAP blocks with indwelling catheters not only compare well with thoracic epidural analgesia, but can be easier to perform and are safer.[60]

Endovascular aneurysm repair

The choice of anesthetic used for an endovascular aneurysm repair (EVAR) is based on the clinical scenario and the patient, surgeon, and anesthesiologist preferences. EVAR can be performed under total intravenous anesthesia, inhalational-based general anesthesia, neuraxial anesthesia, or local anesthesia with conscious sedation (monitored anesthesia care [MAC]). As expected, fewer complications are reported when GA is avoided.[61] Edwards and colleagues[62] analyzed data from the NSQIP database for elective EVAR cases (total 6009 procedures) performed between 2005 and 2008. GA was used in 4868 cases, spinal anesthesia in 419, epidural anesthesia in 331, and local/MAC in 391. Postoperative complications occurred in 11% of patients. GA was associated with an increase in pulmonary morbidity in comparison with spinal or local/MAC anesthesia.

Use of GA was also associated with a 10% increase in length of stay in hospital for GA versus spinal, and a 20% increase for GA versus local/MAC anesthesia. Trends in increased pulmonary morbidity and length of stay were not observed for GA versus epidural anesthesia. Hence, when possible, GA should be avoided. However, GA is unavoidable in patients who cannot lie flat or still, as a motionless operative field is imperative for accurate graft positioning.

Ruptured aneurysms

The IMPROVE trial[63] was a large, randomized clinical trial in which eligible patients with a clinical diagnosis of ruptured abdominal aneurysm were allocated to a strategy of EVAR versus open repair. The impact of time and manner of hospital presentation, fluid volume status, type of anesthesia, type of endovascular repair, and time to aneurysm repair on 30-day mortality were the primary end points. Lowest systolic blood pressure was independently associated with 30-day mortality. The mortality was recorded as 51% among those patients who had a systolic blood pressure lower than 70 mm Hg. Patients who received EVAR under local anesthesia alone had a greatly reduced 30-day mortality compared with those who had GA. As a result, outcomes of ruptured AAAs might be improved by not allowing the minimum blood pressure to fall below the threshold of 70 mm Hg and by promoting a wider use of local anesthesia for EVARs.

Peripheral Artery Procedures

Patients with peripheral vascular disease, even asymptomatic individuals, are at high risk for myocardial infarction, stroke, and death because peripheral vascular disease is a marker of diffuse atherosclerosis. There is no significant difference in amputation-free survival and overall survival between endovascular and open surgical limb salvage procedures. However, an open bypass-first approach (vs angioplasty) is associated with a significant overall survival of 7.3 months and a trend toward amputation-free survival of 5.9 months for patients who survive more than 2 years.[64]

There is considerable controversy regarding the best anesthetic technique for peripheral artery procedures. Singh and colleagues[65] conducted an analysis of the Veteran's Administration NSQIP data and found an increased risk of graft failure, higher incidence of pneumonia, and higher incidence of myocardial infarction with GA in comparison with RA. Conversely, other studies have shown no difference in cardiac and other morbidities between anesthetic techniques.[66]

Several studies have demonstrated an increased graft patency rate with regional anesthesia.[67] In a recent large observational study by Ghanami and colleagues,[68] morbidity and mortality rates were evaluated in RA groups (spinal, epidural, local) and GA groups for lower extremity vascular bypass surgery. The overall morbidity rate was 37%, with no significant difference in the incidence of morbidity (cardiac events, graft failure, postoperative pneumonia, or return to the operating room), mortality, or length of stay between groups. The analysis from pooled data from randomized controlled trials demonstrates that there is no clear evidence in favor of one anesthetic technique over another for peripheral artery procedures, and the choice should be based on clinical judgment.

POSTOPERATIVE MANAGEMENT

A myriad of complications can present during the care of patients undergoing vascular surgery. These complications typically present in the postoperative period and mirror other major organ system complications.[24]

Disposition

Most vascular surgery patients are admitted to the intensive care unit (ICU) following carotid endarterectomies and major abdominal and thoracic vascular procedures. Preexisting comorbidities, surgical and anesthetic techniques, and restrictive policies regarding medication use in specific hospital areas mandate this approach to postoperative care. A prospective study by Melissano and colleagues[69] of patients after carotid endarterectomies demonstrated that selective ICU admission and early postoperative discharge is safe and cost-effective. A case-control study by Lipsett and colleagues[70] suggests a 6- to 8-hour recovery room stay following carotid endarterectomies, allowing selective admission to the ICU.

Factors predictive of ICU admission include a preoperative history of myocardial infarction, hypertension, arrhythmia, and chronic renal failure. This approach has been challenged, citing the increased cost of prolonged recovery room observation and the staffing inefficiencies secondary to uncertain postoperative disposition. Unclear disposition early in the postoperative period can also be confusing for patients and families following major vascular surgery.[71,72]

Care following other vascular procedures has been investigated, and a retrospective study by Bertges and colleagues[73] of patients after open infrarenal abdominal aneurysm repair also demonstrated that selective postoperative non-ICU admissions are safe and cost-effective without compromising quality. Debate will continue as to the best disposition for vascular surgery patients postoperatively. Resource utilization challenges will present opportunities to reevaluate standard pathways, and lead to safe and effective refinements of clinical pathways.

Cardiovascular Issues

Troponin leak

Perioperative myocardial ischemia and infarction remain a consistent risk for patients undergoing vascular surgery. Between 3% and 24% of vascular surgery patients sustain ischemic injuries or postoperative myocardial infarction (MI) based on biochemical markers.[74] Significant morbidity and mortality is associated with perioperative MI. Accordingly, much attention has focused on troponin monitoring postoperatively and the relationship between elevation of troponin levels and outcomes in patients undergoing vascular surgery.

Troponin elevation, in the range of greater than 0.1 to 2 ng/mL, is common following vascular surgery and occurs in 15% of patients.[75] An elevated troponin-T level greater than 0.1 ng/mL is diagnostic for MI.[74] Levels of troponin-T below this diagnostic threshold without electrocardiographic (ECG) or echocardiographic findings consistent with infarction are termed isolated troponin leaks. A small (N = 65) prospective, observational study by Howell and colleagues[76] revealed that 40% of vascular surgery patients have troponin elevations above the lower limit of detection (troponin I >0.0006 μg/L). In addition, two-thirds of these patients demonstrated an isolated troponin leak without signs or symptoms of a perioperative MI.

A meta-analysis by Redfern and colleagues[75] of outcomes following vascular surgery demonstrated a 30-day mortality of 2.3%, 11.6%, and 21.6% based on no elevation, an isolated troponin leak, or perioperative MI, respectively. A cohort study by Landesberg and colleagues[74] demonstrated that cardiac troponin-T levels greater than 0.1 ng/mL predict a 2-fold increase in mortality, independent of common preoperative risk factors in vascular surgery patients; lower levels of elevation (cardiac troponin-T >0.003 ng/mL) independently predict a 1.89-fold increase in mortality.

At present, the ACCF/AHA recommends measurement of postoperative troponins only in patients with ECG changes or pain typical of an acute syndrome (Class I). The measurement of troponins is not well established in patients who are clinically stable following vascular surgery (Class IIb), but recent clinical investigations suggest it may provide some risk stratification.[24,74,75] It can be suggested that routine monitoring of troponins be instituted in vascular surgery patients, and targeted therapy initiated if an elevation is detected.

β-blockers

Patients receiving β-blockers preoperatively should continue to receive them in the perioperative period to prevent cardiac complications or precipitate β-blocker withdrawal. The goal of postoperative β-blockade titration is to obtain a heart rate of 50 to 60 beats per minute.[24] Targeted therapy suggests that each 10-beat-per-minute reduction in heart rate is estimated to reduce the relative risk of cardiac death by 30%.[77] The titrated therapy must avoid hypotension and bradycardia, which can create other significant complications.

Perioperative β-blocker withdrawal should be avoided, and acute withdrawal is associated with an increased risk for angina and MI. The Centers for Medicare and Medicaid Services Surgical Care Improvement Project has expanded the criteria for perioperative β-blocker administration: the first dose should administered on the day of surgery (or within 24 hours preceding skin incision) and the second dose on either postoperative day 1 or postoperative day 2 (http://www.jointcommision.org/assets/1/6/NHQM_v4_3a_PDF_10_2_13.zip).

Neurologic

Various degrees of neurologic changes may occur following vascular surgery. Alterations in mental status may be related to underlying vascular disease, medications, electrolyte imbalances, hypoxia, cardiac disease, or surgical complications. In a retrospective data review by Katznelson and colleagues,[78] postoperative delirium was observed in 22% of 828 vascular surgery patients. Patients who developed delirium were older, and more likely had a history of transient ischemic attack or cerebrovascular accident, CAD, and depression. These patients were also more likely receiving preoperative β-blockers, which doubled the odds of postoperative delirium.

Preoperative statin administration reduced these same odds by 44%. β-Blockers interact with serotonin-sensitive adenylate cyclase systems and melatonin secretion mechanisms, which are part of the neurotransmitter network involved in the pathogenesis of delirium.[79,80] Cerebrovascular accidents can occur following vascular surgery and mirror the occurrence of cardiac events, owing to the similar underlying risk factors for patients undergoing vascular surgery.

Cerebral hyperperfusion syndrome, characterized by hypertension, seizures, and neurologic deficits, can be observed in patients after carotid artery endarterectomies.[81] There is a relationship between a failure of chronically hyperperfused vessels to adapt to increased blood flow and subsequent neurologic dysfunction. Cerebral near-infrared spectroscopy can predict the onset of postoperative cerebral hyperperfusion (**Fig. 1**), with an optimal cutoff value ranging from a 2% to 10% increase in the value of regional oxygen saturation.[82,83] Cerebral hyperperfusion can be prevented with early identification and control of blood pressure (see **Fig. 1**).

Glycemic Control

Glycemic control in the perioperative period has been variably managed for decades. Perioperative management has followed the trend of undermanagement of hyperglycemia in hospitalized patients in general. Multiple factors contribute to practice inertia regarding perioperative hyperglycemia, including: variable study results; hyperglycemia being a secondary concern to other surgical conditions; overwhelming fear of hypoglycemia; and persistent use of ineffective sliding-scale coverage based on historical practice patterns.[84] Sliding-scale insulin coverage has been discounted as an effective management technique to treat hyperglycemia, but perioperative use remains common.[85,86]

Thirty percent of patients presenting for vascular surgery are diabetics, and these patients have an average length of stay in hospital that is 3.5 days longer in comparison with the nondiabetic patient.[87] Studies of glucose levels on the first postoperative day following peripheral vascular surgery demonstrate that they are an independent

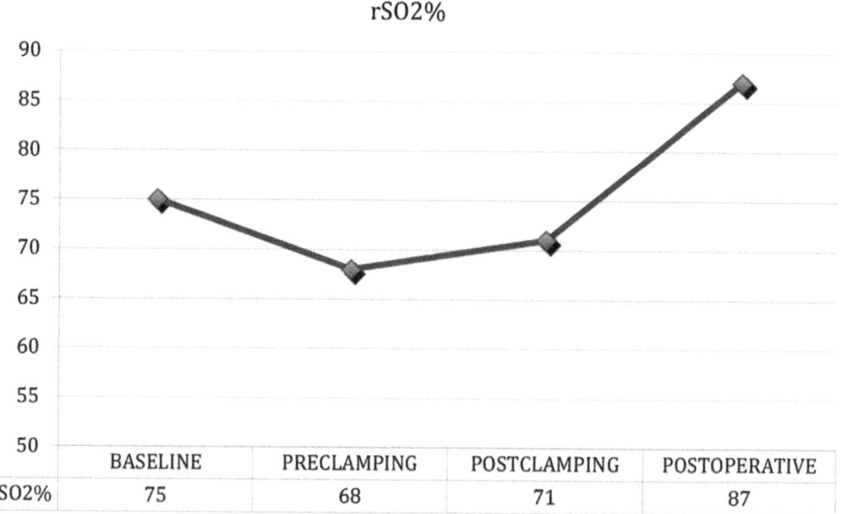

	BASELINE	PRECLAMPING	POSTCLAMPING	POSTOPERATIVE
rSO2%	75	68	71	87

Fig. 1. Hypothetical patient undergoing carotid endarterectomy who develops cerebral hyperperfusion syndrome on postoperative day 1 with severe headache and profound hypertension. rSO2, regional oxygen saturation.

risk factor for infection.[88] Postoperative hyperglycemia occurs in 21% to 34% of patients within 72 hours of surgery.[89] Every 40 mg/dL increase in postoperative glucose measurement leads to a 30% increased risk of postoperative infection and longer length of stay.[90]

A performance improvement project by Najarian and colleagues[87] focused on glycemic control in diabetic patients undergoing vascular surgery. This study demonstrated that implementation of standard intravenous insulin order sets for procedures lasting longer than 2 hours, and a dedicated diabetes nurse educator to facilitate education and implementation of this new pathway, reduced postoperative infections by 19.8%. Despite tighter glycemic control in this group of patients, the rates of hypoglycemia postoperatively did not increase.

Postoperative management of vascular surgery patients with diabetes or stress-induced hyperglycemia should be based on defined guidelines. The American Association of Clinical Endocrinologists and American Diabetes Association issued a consensus statement in 2009[91] regarding inpatient glycemic control, and defined hyperglycemia as a blood glucose value greater than 140 mg/dL and hypoglycemia as a blood glucose value less than 70 mg/dL. Treatment of hyperglycemia in the ICU should begin with an intravenous insulin infusion with a starting threshold no higher than 180 mg/dL. Intravenous insulin should be used to maintain blood glucose values between 140 and 180 mg/dL, although some benefit may be realized with lower target levels.

In the non-ICU patient population, premeal glucose targets should be less than 140 mg/dL in conjunction with random blood glucose levels less than 180 mg/dL. Scheduled subcutaneous administration of insulin is preferred for achieving and maintaining glycemic control in non-ICU patients. The 3 recommended components of therapy include a basal, nutritional, and supplemental (correction) element to the insulin therapy. Attention should focus on eliminating sliding-scale insulin coverage, which has been proved to be ineffective.

Supplemental (correction) insulin dosing should be used to treat blood glucose levels that are off-target between the scheduled insulin. An insulin infusion may become necessary to provide tighter control for patients who remain hyperglycemic despite close attention to dosing in the 3-component format. The use of oral noninsulin agents to treat blood glucose is not indicated for hospitalized patients because of the potential complications.

Greater attention needs to be focused on perioperative glycemic control to optimize outcomes. Hospital-based improvement processes focused exclusively on inpatient glycemic control are cost-effective and should be replicated at more institutions.[92] Physician and nurse champions, staff education, protocols, order sets, and system-based improvement processes are needed to combat this persistent issue.

Renal

Patients undergoing vascular procedures are at risk for renal failure secondary to associated medical conditions such as hypertension, peripheral arterial disease, hyperlipidemia, diabetes, and smoking. Surgical risk factors include cross-clamping of the aorta and the administration of radiographic dye. Kheterpal and colleagues[93] observed 15,102 patients undergoing major noncardiac surgery over a 3-year period. These patients had a preoperative creatinine clearance greater than 80 mL/min. The incidence of acute renal failure (creatinine clearance decreasing to <50 mL/min postoperatively) was 0.8% and the need for dialysis was 0.1%. Preoperative predictors of renal failure included age, emergency surgery, liver disease, body mass index, high-risk surgery, peripheral vascular disease, and chronic obstructive pulmonary disease.

Intraoperative risk factors included use of a vasopressor infusion, total vasopressor dose administered, and diuretic administration. Acute renal failure following noncardiac surgery increased 30-, 60-, and 365-day all-cause mortality, with vascular surgery patients accounting for 17% of those who developed acute renal failure. Studies specific to vascular surgical procedures also demonstrate a relationship between increased mortality and acute renal failure following emergency vascular surgery.[94]

Endovascular approaches to elective AAA repair may have lower rates of postoperative acute renal failure, although the literature varies on this issue owing to differences in study design.[95,96] Postoperative care should focus on adequate renal perfusion to prevent further insult to the kidney following major vascular surgery.

Pain Management

Comprehensive perioperative pain management is important to facilitate compassionate and effective postoperative care. Research identifies inadequate postoperative pain therapy as a significant issue in health care. A small survey study (N = 17) of ICU patients by Whipple and colleagues[97] demonstrated that perceptions regarding quality of pain control differ between members of the care team and patients. This study found that 72% of trauma ICU patients reported feeling moderate to severe pain, whereas resident physicians and nurses considered that adequate pain control was being achieved in these same patients 95% and 81% of the time, respectively. This discrepancy is important because decreasing or eliminating the physiologic responses to surgical trauma can lead to improved short-term and long-term outcomes.

The effective treatment of acute surgical pain may decrease the likelihood of a patient developing a chronic pain syndrome. The incidence of phantom limb pain following amputations varies from 30% to 81%.[98] Postoperative factors leading to chronic pain following an amputation include preoperative limb pain, chemotherapy use, and persistent stump pain at 1 week. Use of local anesthesia either at the nerve-sheath level or via an epidural catheter has led to conflicting results with regard to decreasing chronic pain following amputations.[98]

Intravenous opioids are the cornerstones of the treatment of surgical pain, but are associated with well-known complications including nausea and vomiting, respiratory depression, and decreased gastrointestinal motility. The increase in prevalence of obesity and sleep apnea has also led to an increased risk for respiratory complications in patients receiving intravenous opioids. Concerns over side effects, especially potential respiratory depression and hypotension, continue to be a barrier to adequate pain management in the postoperative period.[97]

Multimodal pain therapy that includes nonopioid strategies is necessary to improve the efficacy of pain relief and decrease the risk of side effects and complications. Nonopioid agents such as acetaminophen and nonsteriodal anti-inflammatory drugs (NSAIDs) have been evaluated for the management of mild to moderate pain. Two recent meta-analyses of the literature on a variety of surgical procedures suggest that the use of acetaminophen, propacetamol, and/or paracetamol improves pain control and reduces opiate consumption, although these medications unfortunately do not decrease opiate-related complications.[99,100]

NSAIDs have analgesic, anti-inflammatory, and antipyretic effects, and when used concomitantly may decrease postoperative morphine consumption by 30% to 50%.[101] Marret and colleagues[102] demonstrated in a meta-analysis that there can be a reduction in certain opioid-related complications with NSAID use. These investigators found that postoperative opioid-related nausea and vomiting decreased by 29%, but found no significant effects on respiratory depression. Concerns over bleeding, gastrointestinal ulceration, renal injury, cardiac ischemia/infarction, stroke, and bone and wound healing have limited the widespread utilization of these agents postoperatively.[101]

Other multimodal adjuncts include, but are not limited to, ketamine, pregabalin, and gabapentin. Ketamine, an *N*-methyl-D-aspartate antagonist, has been used in different treatment pathways perioperatively. Low-dose ketamine (0.1–0.2 mg/kg intravenously) reduces opioid consumption and decreases opioid-related complications postoperatively.[103] Various dosing regimens have been evaluated in attempts to decrease postoperative pain, including single intraoperative doses, continuous postoperative infusions, or a combination of ketamine with intravenous opioid patient-controlled analgesia. No single standard has been defined.

The γ-aminobutyric acid analogues, pregabalin and gabapentin, although not marketed for postoperative pain, have been shown to decrease pain following orthopedic and laparoscopic procedures, and cesarean sections. Pregabalin has antihyperalgesic properties. A meta-analysis by Zhang and colleagues[104] of 11 randomized controlled trials demonstrated that cumulative 24-hour opioid consumption is decreased when pregabalin is administered, even though no change is noted in postoperative pain intensity scores on a visual analogue scale. A preoperative dose of less than 300 mg is related to opioid-sparing effects while doses greater than 300 mg produce an even larger decrease in postoperative opioid consumption. Pregabalin use reduces opioid-related adverse effects, including nausea and vomiting, but does increase the risk of visual disturbances postoperatively.

Finally, there is continued interest in the use of regional anesthesia, including both neuraxial and peripheral nerve blocks, to treat perioperative pain. Concerns regarding newer antiplatelet therapies that provide cardiovascular and neurologic benefits may preclude safe administration of regional anesthesia.

SUMMARY

Being well informed on updated national guidelines is imperative in the administration of appropriate care to patients undergoing vascular surgery. The changing landscape of this surgical field has helped to improve the outcome of these patients, but due care and attention is needed to provide the best perioperative medical management.

REFERENCES

1. Fleisher LA, Beckman JA, Brown KA, et al. ACC/AHA 2007 Guidelines on Perioperative Cardiovascular Evaluation and Care for Noncardiac Surgery: a report of the American College of Cardiology/American Heart Association Task Force on Practice Guidelines (Writing Committee to Revise the 2002 Guidelines on Perioperative Cardiovascular Evaluation for Noncardiac Surgery): developed in Collaboration with the American Society of Echocardiography, American Society of Nuclear Cardiology, Heart Rhythm Society, Society of Cardiovascular Anesthesiologists, Society for Cardiovascular Angiography and Interventions, Society for Vascular Medicine and Biology, and Society for Vascular Surgery. Circulation 2007;116(17):e418–99.
2. Omar HR, Mangar D, Camporesi EM. Preoperative cardiac evaluation of the vascular surgery patient–an anesthesia perspective. Vasc Endovascular Surg 2012;46(3):201–11.
3. Hertzer NR, Young JR, Kramer JR, et al. Routine coronary angiography prior to elective aortic reconstruction: results of selective myocardial revascularization in patients with peripheral vascular disease. Arch Surg 1979;114(11):1336–44.

4. Bauer SM, Cayne NS, Veith FJ. New developments in the preoperative evaluation and perioperative management of coronary artery disease in patients undergoing vascular surgery. J Vasc Surg 2010;51(1):242–51.
5. Virgilio C, Wall DB, Ephraim L, et al. An abnormal dipyridamole thallium/sestamibi fails to predict long-term cardiac events in vascular surgery patients. Ann Vasc Surg 2001;15(2):267–71.
6. Garcia S, Moritz TE, Ward HB, et al. Usefulness of revascularization of patients with multivessel coronary artery disease before elective vascular surgery for abdominal aortic and peripheral occlusive disease. Am J Cardiol 2008;102(7): 809–13.
7. McFalls EO, Ward HB, Moritz TE, et al. Coronary-artery revascularization before elective major vascular surgery. N Engl J Med 2004;351(27):2795–804.
8. Stone DH, Goodney PP, Schanzer A, et al. Clopidogrel is not associated with major bleeding complications during peripheral arterial surgery. J Vasc Surg 2011;54(3):779–84.
9. Saadeh C, Sfeir J. Discontinuation of preoperative clopidogrel is unnecessary in peripheral arterial surgery. J Vasc Surg 2013;58(6):1586–92.
10. Paty PS, Darling C III, Chang BB, et al. Repair of large abdominal aortic aneurysm should be performed early after coronary artery bypass surgery. J Vasc Surg 2000;31(2):253–9.
11. Cowie B. Focused cardiovascular ultrasound performed by anesthesiologists in the perioperative period: feasible and alters patient management. J Cardiothorac Vasc Anesth 2009;23(4):450–6.
12. Cowie B. Three years' experience of focused cardiovascular ultrasound in the peri-operative period. Anaesthesia 2011;66(4):268–73.
13. Fleisher LA, Beckman JA, Brown KA, et al. 2009 ACCF/AHA focused update on perioperative beta blockade incorporated into the ACC/AHA 2007 guidelines on perioperative cardiovascular evaluation and care for noncardiac surgery: a report of the American College of Cardiology foundation/American Heart Association Task Force on practice guidelines. Circulation 2009;120(21): e169–276.
14. Shammash JB, Trost JC, Gold JM, et al. Perioperative beta-blocker withdrawal and mortality in vascular surgical patients. Am Heart J 2001;141(1):148–53.
15. POISE Study Group, Devereaux PJ, Yang H, et al. Effects of extended-release metoprolol succinate in patients undergoing non-cardiac surgery (POISE Trial): a randomised controlled trial. Lancet 2008;371(9627):1839–47.
16. Wiesbauer F, Schlager O, Domanovits H, et al. Perioperative Beta-blockers for preventing surgery-related mortality and morbidity: a systematic review and meta-analysis. Anesth Analg 2007;104(1):27–41.
17. Flu WJ, van Kuijk JP, Chonchol M, et al. Timing of pre-operative beta-blocker treatment in vascular surgery patients: influence on post-operative outcome. J Am Coll Cardiol 2010;56(23):1922–9.
18. Poldermans D, Boersma E, Bax JJ, et al. The effect of bisoprolol on perioperative mortality and myocardial infarction in high-risk patients undergoing vascular surgery. Dutch echocardiographic cardiac risk evaluation applying stress echocardiography study group. N Engl J Med 1999;341(24):1789–94.
19. Wallace AW, Au S, Cason BA. Perioperative beta-blockade: atenolol is associated with reduced mortality when compared to metoprolol. Anesthesiology 2011;114(4):824–36.
20. Mashour GA, Sharifpour M, Freundlich RE, et al. Perioperative metoprolol and risk of stroke after noncardiac surgery. Anesthesiology 2013;119(6):1340–6.

21. Foex P, Sear JW. II. Beta-blockers and cardiac protection: 5 yr on from POISE. Br J Anaesth 2014;112(2):206–10.
22. Hirsch AT, Haskal ZJ, Hertzer NR, et al. ACC/AHA 2005 Practice Guidelines for the management of patients with peripheral arterial disease (lower extremity, renal, mesenteric, and abdominal aortic): a collaborative report from the American Association for Vascular Surgery/Society for Vascular Surgery, Society for Cardiovascular Angiography and Interventions, Society for Vascular Medicine and Biology, Society of Interventional Radiology, and the ACC/AHA Task Force on Practice Guidelines (Writing Committee to Develop Guidelines for the Management of Patients with Peripheral Arterial Disease): Endorsed by the American Association of Cardiovascular and Pulmonary Rehabilitation; National Heart, Lung, and Blood Institute; Society for Vascular Nursing; TransAtlantic Inter-Society Consensus; and Vascular Disease Foundation. Circulation 2006; 113(11):e463–654.
23. Railton CJ, Wolpin J, Lam-McCulloch J, et al. Renin-angiotensin blockade is associated with increased mortality after vascular surgery. Can J Anaesth 2010;57(8):736–44.
24. Fleisher LA, Beckman JA, Brown KA, et al. 2009 ACCF/AHA focused update on perioperative beta blockade incorporated into the ACC/AHA 2007 guidelines on perioperative cardiovascular evaluation and care for noncardiac surgery. J Am Coll Cardiol 2009;54(22):e13–118.
25. 2011 Writing Group Members, 2005 Writing Committee Members, ACCF/AHA Task Force Members. 2011 ACCF/AHA focused update of the guideline for the management of patients with peripheral artery disease (updating the 2005 guideline): a report of the American College of Cardiology Foundation/American Heart Association Task Force on practice guidelines. Circulation 2011;124(18):2020–45.
26. Woehlck HJ, Connolly LA, Cinquegrani MP, et al. Acute smoking increases ST depression in humans during general anesthesia. Anesth Analg 1999;89(4): 856–60.
27. Barrera R, Shi W, Amar D, et al. Smoking and timing of cessation: impact on pulmonary complications after thoracotomy. Chest 2005;127(6):1977–83.
28. Brott TG, Halperin JL, Abbara S, et al. 2011 ASA/ACCF/AHA/AANN/AANS/ACR/ASNR/CNS/SAIP/SCAI/SIR/SNIS/SVM/SVS guideline on the management of patients with extracranial carotid and vertebral artery disease: executive summary. A report of the American College of Cardiology Foundation/American Heart Association Task Force on Practice Guidelines, and the American Stroke Association, American Association of Neuroscience Nurses, American Association of Neurological Surgeons, American College of Radiology, American Society of Neuroradiology, Congress of Neurological Surgeons, Society of Atherosclerosis Imaging and Prevention, Society for Cardiovascular Angiography and Interventions, Society of Interventional Radiology, Society of NeuroInterventional Surgery, Society for Vascular Medicine, and Society for Vascular Surgery. Circulation 2011;124(4):489–532.
29. Grines CL, Bonow RO, Casey DE Jr, et al. Prevention of premature discontinuation of dual antiplatelet therapy in patients with coronary artery stents: a science advisory from the American Heart Association, American College of Cardiology, Society for Cardiovascular Angiography and Interventions, American College of Surgeons, and American Dental Association, with Representation from the American College of Physicians. Circulation 2007;115(6):813–8.
30. American Society of Anesthesiologists Committee on Standards and Practice Parameters. Practice alert for the perioperative management of patients with

coronary artery stents: a report by the American Society of Anesthesiologists Committee on Standards and Practice Parameters. Anesthesiology 2009; 110(1):22–3.
31. Smith SC Jr, Benjamin EJ, Bonow RO, et al. AHA/ACCF secondary prevention and risk reduction therapy for patients with coronary and other atherosclerotic vascular disease: 2011 update: a guideline from the American Heart Association and American College of Cardiology Foundation. Circulation 2011; 124(22):2458–73.
32. Horlocker TT, Wedel DJ, Rowlingson JC, et al. Regional anesthesia in the patient receiving antithrombotic or thrombolytic therapy: American Society of Regional Anesthesia and Pain Medicine Evidence-Based Guidelines (Third Edition). Reg Anesth Pain Med 2010;35(1):64–101.
33. Gayle JA, Kaye AD, Kaye AM, et al. Anticoagulants: newer ones, mechanisms, and perioperative updates. Anesthesiol clin 2010;28(4):667–79.
34. Ang-Lee MK, Moss J, Yuan CS. Herbal medicines and perioperative care. JAMA 2001;286(2):208–16.
35. The Emerging Risk Factors Collaboration, et al. Diabetes mellitus, fasting blood glucose concentration, and risk of vascular disease: a collaborative meta-analysis of 102 prospective studies. Lancet 2010;375(9733):2215–22.
36. Avogaro A, Albiero M, Menegazzo L, et al. Endothelial dysfunction in diabetes: the role of reparatory mechanisms. Diabetes Care 2011;34(Suppl 2):S285–90.
37. O'Sullivan CJ, Hynes N, Mahendran B, et al. Haemoglobin A1c (HbA1C) in non-diabetic and diabetic vascular patients. Is HbA1C an independent risk factor and predictor of adverse outcome? Eur J Vasc Endovasc Surg 2006;32(2):188–97.
38. McGirt MJ, Woodworth GF, Brooke BS, et al. Hyperglycemia independently increases the risk of perioperative stroke, myocardial infarction, and death after carotid endarterectomy. Neurosurgery 2006;58(6):1066–73 [discussion: 1066–73].
39. van Kuijk JP, Schouten O, Flu WJ, et al. Perioperative blood glucose monitoring and control in major vascular surgery patients. Eur J Vasc Endovasc Surg 2009; 38(5):627–34.
40. Campos JH. Noncardiac pulmonary, endocrine, and renal preoperative evaluation of the vascular surgical patient. Anesthesiol Clin North America 2004;22(2): 209–22, vi.
41. Manley AM, Reck SE. Patients with vascular disease. Med Clin North Am 2013; 97(6):1077–93.
42. Scheeren TW, Wiesenack C, Gerlach H, et al. Goal-directed intraoperative fluid therapy guided by stroke volume and its variation in high-risk surgical patients: a prospective randomized multicentre study. J Clin Monit Comput 2013;27(3): 225–33.
43. Romagnoli S, Ricci Z, Romano SM, et al. FloTrac/Vigileo (TM) (third generation) and MostCare (®)/PRAM versus echocardiography for cardiac output estimation in vascular surgery. J Cardiothorac Vasc Anesth 2013;27(6):1114–21.
44. McArdle GT, Price G, Lewis A, et al. Positive fluid balance is associated with complications after elective open infrarenal abdominal aortic aneurysm repair. Eur J Vasc Endovasc Surg 2007;34(5):522–7.
45. Toomtong P, Suksompong S. Intravenous fluids for abdominal aortic surgery. Cochrane Database Syst Rev 2010;(1):CD000991. http://dx.doi.org/10.1002/14651858.CD000991.
46. Bunn F, Trivedi D. Colloid solutions for fluid resuscitation. Cochrane Database Syst Rev 2012;(7):CD001319.

47. Mutter TC, Ruth CA, Dart AB. Hydroxyethyl starch (HES) versus other fluid therapies: effects on kidney function. Cochrane Database Syst Rev 2013;(7):CD007594.
48. Le Manach Y, Collins GS, Ibanez C, et al. Impact of perioperative bleeding on the protective effect of beta-blockers during infrarenal aortic reconstruction. Anesthesiology 2012;117(6):1203–11.
49. Schechter MA, Shortell CK, Scarborough JE. Regional versus general anesthesia for carotid endarterectomy: the American College of Surgeons National Surgical Quality Improvement Program perspective. Surgery 2012;152(3): 309–14.
50. GALA Trial Collaborative Group, Lewis SC, Warlow CP, et al. General anaesthesia versus local anaesthesia for carotid surgery (GALA): a multicentre, randomised controlled trial. Lancet 2008;372(9656):2132–42.
51. Forssell C, Takolander R, Bergqvist D, et al. Local versus general anaesthesia in carotid surgery. A prospective, randomised study. Eur J Vasc Surg 1989;3(6): 503–9.
52. Murie JA, John TG, Morris PJ. Carotid endarterectomy in Great Britain and Ireland: practice between 1984 and 1992. Br J Surg 1994;81(6):827–31.
53. Browse NL, Russell RR. Carotid endarterectomy and the Javid shunt: the early results of 215 consecutive operations for transient ischaemic attacks. Br J Surg 1984;71(1):53–7.
54. Santamaria G, Britti RD, Tescione M, et al. Comparison between local and general anaesthesia for carotid endarterectomy. A retrospective analysis. Minerva Anestesiol 2004;70(11):771–8.
55. Pandit JJ, Satya-Krishna R, Gration P. Superficial or deep cervical plexus block for carotid endarterectomy: a systematic review of complications. Br J Anaesth 2007;99(2):159–69.
56. Marcucci G, Siani A, Accrocca F, et al. Preserved consciousness in general anesthesia during carotid endarterectomy: a six-year experience. Interact Cardiovasc Thorac Surg 2012;13(6):601–5.
57. Nishimori M, Low JH, Zheng H, et al. Epidural pain relief versus systemic opioid-based pain relief for abdominal aortic surgery. Cochrane Database Syst Rev 2012;(7):CD005059.
58. Licker M, Christoph E, Cartier V, et al. Impact of anesthesia technique on the incidence of major complications after open aortic abdominal surgery: a cohort study. J Clin Anesth 2013;25(4):296–308.
59. Kheterpal S, Tremper KK, Heung M, et al. Development and validation of an acute kidney injury risk index for patients undergoing general surgery: results from a national data set. Anesthesiology 2009;110(3):505–15.
60. Niraj G, Kelkar A, Jeyapalan I, et al. Comparison of analgesic efficacy of subcostal transversus abdominis plane blocks with epidural analgesia following upper abdominal surgery. Anaesthesia 2011;66(6):465–71.
61. Verhoeven EL, Prins TR, van den Dungen JJ, et al. Endovascular repair of acute AAAs under local anesthesia with bifurcated endografts: a feasibility study. J Endovasc Ther 2002;9(6):729–35.
62. Edwards MS, Andrews JS, Edwards AF, et al. Results of endovascular aortic aneurysm repair with general, regional, and local/monitored anesthesia care in the American College of Surgeons National Surgical Quality Improvement Program database. J Vasc Surg 2011;54(5):1273–82.
63. IMPROVE Trial Investigators. Observations from the IMPROVE trial concerning the clinical care of patients with ruptured abdominal aortic aneurysm. Br J Surg 2014;101(3):216–24.

64. Adam DJ, Beard JD, Cleveland T, et al. Bypass versus angioplasty in severe ischaemia of the leg (basil): multicentre, randomised controlled trial. Lancet 2005;366(9501):1925–34.
65. Singh N, Sidawy AN, Dezee K, et al. The effects of the type of anesthesia on outcomes of lower extremity infrainguinal bypass. J Vasc Surg 2006;44(5):964–8 [discussion: 968–70].
66. Pierce ET, Pomposelli FB Jr, Stanley GD, et al. Anesthesia type does not influence early graft patency or limb salvage rates of lower extremity arterial bypass. J Vasc Surg 1997;25(2):226–32 [discussion: 232–3].
67. Perler BA, Christopherson R, Rosenfeld BA, et al. The influence of anesthetic method on infrainguinal bypass graft patency: a closer look. Am Surg 1995; 61(9):784–9.
68. Ghanami RJ, Hurie J, Andrews JS, et al. Anesthesia-based evaluation of outcomes of lower-extremity vascular bypass procedures. Ann Vasc Surg 2013; 27(2):199–207.
69. Melissano G, Castellano R, Mazzitelli S, et al. Safe and cost-effective approach to carotid surgery. Eur J Vasc Endovasc Surg 1997;14(3):164–9.
70. Lipsett PA, Tierney S, Gordon TA, et al. Carotid endarterectomy–is intensive care unit care necessary? J Vasc Surg 1994;20(3):403–9 [discussion: 409–10].
71. Ross SD, Tribble CG, Parrino PE, et al. Intensive care is cost-effective in carotid endarterectomy. Cardiovasc Surg 2000;8(1):41–6.
72. Teplick R, Caldera DL, Gilbert JP, et al. Benefit of elective intensive care admission after certain operations. Anesth Analg 1983;62(6):572–7.
73. Bertges DJ, Rhee RY, Muluk SC, et al. Is routine use of the intensive care unit after elective infrarenal abdominal aortic aneurysm repair necessary? J Vasc Surg 2000;32(4):634–42.
74. Landesberg G, Shatz V, Akopnik I, et al. Association of cardiac troponin, CK-MB, and postoperative myocardial ischemia with long-term survival after major vascular surgery. J Am Coll Cardiol 2003;42(9):1547–54.
75. Redfern G, Rodseth RN, Biccard BM. Outcomes in vascular surgical patients with isolated postoperative troponin leak: a meta-analysis. Anaesthesia 2011; 66(7):604–10.
76. Howell SJ, Thompson JP, Nimmo AF, et al. Relationship between perioperative troponin elevation and other indicators of myocardial injury in vascular surgery patients. Br J Anaesth 2006;96(3):303–9.
77. Cucherat M. Quantitative relationship between resting heart rate reduction and magnitude of clinical benefits in post-myocardial infarction: a meta-regression of randomized clinical trials. Eur Heart J 2007;28(24):3012–9.
78. Katznelson R, Djaiani G, Mitsakakis N, et al. Delirium following vascular surgery: increased incidence with preoperative beta-blocker administration. Can J Anaesth 2009;56(11):793–801.
79. Brismar K, Hylander B, Eliasson K, et al. Melatonin secretion related to side-effects of beta-blockers from the central nervous system. Acta Med Scand 1988;223(6):525–30.
80. van der Mast RC, Fekkes D. Serotonin and amino acids: partners in delirium pathophysiology? Semin Clin Neuropsychiatry 2000;5(2):125–31.
81. van Mook WN, Rennenberg RJ, Schurink GW, et al. Cerebral hyperperfusion syndrome. Lancet Neurol 2005;4(12):877–88.
82. Ogasawara K, Konno H, Yukawa H, et al. Transcranial regional cerebral oxygen saturation monitoring during carotid endarterectomy as a predictor of postoperative hyperperfusion. Neurosurgery 2003;53(2):309–14 [discussion: 314–5].

83. Pennekamp CW, Immink RV, den Ruijter HM, et al. Near-infrared spectroscopy can predict the onset of cerebral hyperperfusion syndrome after carotid endarterectomy. Cerebrovasc Dis 2012;34(4):314–21.
84. Umpierrez G, Maynard G. Glycemic chaos (not glycemic control) still the rule for inpatient care: how do we stop the insanity? J Hosp Med 2006;1(3):141–4.
85. Gill G, MacFarlane I. Are sliding-scale insulin regimens a recipe for diabetic instability? Lancet 1997;349(9064):1555.
86. Knecht LA, Gauthier SM, Castro JC, et al. Diabetes care in the hospital: is there clinical inertia? J Hosp Med 2006;1(3):151–60.
87. Najarian J, Swavely D, Wilson E, et al. Improving outcomes for diabetic patients undergoing vascular surgery. Diabetes Spectrum 2005;18(1):53–60.
88. Vriesendorp TM, Morelis Q, Devries J, et al. Early post-operative glucose levels are an independent risk factor for infection after peripheral vascular surgery. A retrospective study. Eur J Vasc Endovasc Surg 2004;28(5):520–5.
89. Mahid SS, Polk HC Jr, Lewis JN, et al. Opportunities for improved performance in surgical specialty practice. Ann Surg 2008;247(2):380–8.
90. Ramos M, Khalpey Z, Lipsitz S, et al. Relationship of perioperative hyperglycemia and postoperative infections in patients who undergo general and vascular surgery. Ann Surg 2008;248(4):585–91.
91. Moghissi ES, Korytkowski MT, DiNardo M, et al. American Association of Clinical Endocrinologists and American Diabetes Association consensus statement on inpatient glycemic control. Diabetes care 2009;32(6):1119–31.
92. Krinsley JS, Jones RL. Cost analysis of intensive glycemic control in critically ill adult patients. Chest 2006;129(3):644–50.
93. Kheterpal S, Tremper KK, Englesbe MJ, et al. Predictors of postoperative acute renal failure after noncardiac surgery in patients with previously normal renal function. Anesthesiology 2007;107(6):892–902.
94. Barratt J, Parajasingam R, Sayers RD, et al. Outcome of acute renal failure following surgical repair of ruptured abdominal aortic aneurysms. Eur J Vasc Endovasc Surg 2000;20(2):163–8.
95. Hua HT, Cambria RP, Chuang SK, et al. Early outcomes of endovascular versus open abdominal aortic aneurysm repair in the national surgical quality improvement program-private sector (NSQIP-PS). J Vasc Surg 2005;41(3):382–9.
96. Wald R, Waikar SS, Liangos O, et al. Acute renal failure after endovascular vs open repair of abdominal aortic aneurysm. J Vasc Surg 2006;43(3):460–6 [discussion: 466].
97. Whipple JK, Lewis KS, Quebbeman EJ, et al. Analysis of pain management in critically ill patients. Pharmacotherapy 1995;15(5):592–9.
98. Perkins FM, Kehlet H. Chronic pain as an outcome of surgery. A review of predictive factors. Anesthesiology 2000;93(4):1123–33.
99. McNicol ED, Tzortzopoulou A, Cepeda MS, et al. Single-dose intravenous paracetamol or propacetamol for prevention or treatment of postoperative pain: a systematic review and meta-analysis. Br J Anaesth 2011;106(6):764–75.
100. Remy C, Marret E, Bonnet F. Effects of acetaminophen on morphine side-effects and consumption after major surgery: meta-analysis of randomized controlled trials. Br J Anaesth 2005;94(4):505–13.
101. Beaulieu P. Non-opioid strategies for acute pain management. Can J Anaesth 2007;54(6):481–5.
102. Marret E, Kurdi O, Zufferey P, et al. Effects of nonsteroidal antiinflammatory drugs on patient-controlled analgesia morphine side effects: meta-analysis of randomized controlled trials. Anesthesiology 2005;102(6):1249–60.

103. Bell RF, Dahl JB, Moore RA, et al. Peri-operative ketamine for acute post-operative pain: a quantitative and qualitative systematic review (Cochrane review). Acta Anaesthesiol Scand 2005;49(10):1405–28.
104. Zhang J, Ho KY, Wang Y. Efficacy of pregabalin in acute postoperative pain: a meta-analysis. Br J Anaesth 2011;106(4):454–62. http://dx.doi.org/10.1093/bja/aer027.

Regional Anesthesia for Vascular Surgery

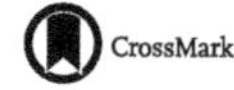

James Flaherty, MD*, Jean-Louis Horn, MD, Ryan Derby, MD, MPH

KEYWORDS

- Regional anesthesia • Cervical plexus blockade • Brachial plexus blockade
- Transversus abdominis plane block • Lumbar and lumbosacral plexus blockade
- Vascular surgery • Perioperative outcomes

KEY POINTS

- Cervical plexus blockade can be performed safely as the primary anesthetic in patients undergoing carotid endarterectomy.
- Medically complex patients undergoing open abdominal aortic aneurysm (AAA) repair are at significant risk of postoperative complications and systemic side effects from intravenous analgesia.
- Endovascular repair of abdominal aortic aneurysms allows repair of AAA in patients too medically complex for open repair.
- Regional anesthesia for lower extremity bypass may reduce graft failure rate, and prolonged perineural infusion may reduce phantom limb pains in lower extremity amputation.
- Regional anesthesia produces sympathectomy, leading to venodilation, improving fistula planning and potentially increasing postoperative fistula flow.

INTRODUCTION

The patient population undergoing vascular surgery presents a challenge because of systemic comorbidities, including hypertension, diabetes mellitus, congestive heart failure, and renal impairment. Ninety-two percent of patients with peripheral vascular disease have angiographic evidence of coronary artery disease (CAD), and likely a high rate of CAD exists in patients with carotid and abdominal aortic atherosclerotic disease. Some degree of myocardial ischemia may occur in up to 28% of patients undergoing major vascular surgery.[1] In addition, the high prevalence of active smoking in the patient population increases the risk of perioperative pulmonary complications.[2] Regional anesthesia is appealing for surgical anesthesia and postoperative pain management in these patients to decrease side effects of systemic medication administration, avoid endotracheal intubation, and reduce hemodynamic fluctuations from sympathetic activation.

Stanford Hospital and Clinics, 300 Pasteur Drive, Room H3580, Stanford, CA 94305, USA
* Corresponding author.
E-mail address: jmflaher@stanford.edu

Anesthesiology Clin 32 (2014) 639–659
http://dx.doi.org/10.1016/j.anclin.2014.05.002 **anesthesiology.theclinics.com**
1932-2275/14/$ – see front matter

Procedures from arteriovenous fistula (AVF) creation to open AAA repair have been performed safely under regional anesthesia alone or as combined general-regional anesthesia. Still, the risks and benefits of regional anesthesia for a particular patient must be carefully weighed. A fundamental concern with the use of regional anesthesia for vascular surgery is the high rate of anticoagulant use in these patients. **Table 1** summarizes the 2010 American Society of Regional Anesthesia (ASRA) guidelines for anticoagulation management for patients receiving neuraxial anesthesia. There is risk of bleeding and epidural hematoma formation with both insertion and removal of an epidural catheter. In addition, ASRA suggests following these guidelines for the performance of deep plexus or peripheral nerve blockade.[3] These guidelines state that it is safe to administer intravenous heparin to the vascular surgery patient as little as 1 hour after performance of regional anesthesia.

Several newer anticoagulants (GIIb-IIIa inhibitors, thrombin inhibitors, rivaroxiban, argatroban, or fondaparinux) have shown great efficacy and represent new challenges for the use of regional anesthesia. ASRA is preparing new regional anesthesia guidelines for their use.

Table 1
ASRA guidelines for nerve anticoagulant management before nerve blockade

Anticoagulant[a]	Discontinuation Before Neuraxial Block/After Removal of Catheter	Administration After Neuraxial Block/Catheter Withdrawal
Unfractionated heparin, subcutaneous		
≤5000 units twice a day for ≤3 d	No contraindication	1 h
≤5000 units for ≥4 d	Assess platelet count	1 h
>10,000 units twice a day or any 3 times a day dosing	Safety not established	Safety not established
Unfractionated Heparin, Intravenous	4 h, consider ACT	1 h
Low-Molecular-Weight Heparin		
Prophylactic dose/single daily dosing	12 h	6–8 h after insertion, 2 h after removal
Therapeutic dose/twice daily dosing	24 h	Indwelling catheter not recommended. Hold dose 24 h before block placement, remove catheter at least 2 h before administration
Warfarin	4–5 d and normalization of INR for insertion, INR <1.5 for removal	Can be initiated, INR should not exceed 1.5 with indwelling catheter
Nonsteroidal antiinflammatory drugs/aspirin	No contraindication	No contraindication
Ticlopidine	14 d	No recommendation
Clopidogrel	7 d	No recommendation
Herbals (gingko, garlic, ginseng)	No contraindication	No contraindication

Abbreviations: ACT, activated clotting time; INR, international normalized ratio.
[a] Refers to single modality of anticoagulation. Multimodal anticoagulation and regional anesthesia safety not well established.

In this article, regional anesthesia for carotid endarterectomy (CEA), abdominal aortic aneurysm (AAA) repair, AVF formation, lower extremity bypass surgery, and lower extremity amputation are discussed.

GENERAL CONCEPTS FOR BLOCK PERFORMANCE

Patient Preparation

Before performing all blocks, a thorough review of the patient's history, focusing on use of anticoagulant medications, existing neuropathies, and concomitant respiratory disease, should be obtained. An international normalized ratio (INR) should be reviewed if the patient is taking warfarin or suffering from liver disease. Risks, benefits, and alternatives to regional anesthesia are discussed with patient. Intravenous access should be established, and standard monitors applied. Apply oxygen by nasal cannula or face mask. Light sedation can be administered to decrease patient anxiety.

Avoiding Complications

The complications listed in **Table 2** are common to all blocks covered in this article. Block-specific complications are addressed in each individual section.

CEA

Regional anesthesia was originally described as the primary anesthetic for CEA in 1962[4] as an effort to improve neurologic monitoring during carotid cross-clamping. Since then, regional anesthesia has been associated with decreased risk of stroke[5,6] and immediate postoperative cognitive dysfunction,[7] myocardial infarction (MI),[8,9] perioperative hemodynamic instability and vasopressor use,[10–12] and postoperative opioid use.[13] Other investigations have shown that regional anesthesia reduces the rate of shunt placement,[11] operating time,[11,14] and hospital length of stay.[8] A systematic review by Guay[15] in 2007 analyzed prospective and retrospective trials comparing regional and general anesthesia and found statistically significant reductions in stroke, death, and MI. However, there remains debate about optimal anesthetic technique for CEA, given the retrospective nature of most data included in this study.

The GALA (General Anesthetic Versus Local Anesthetic for Carotid Surgery) trial,[12] the premiere prospective trial, enrolled 3526 patients but failed to show a statistically significant improvement in stroke, MI, or death with combined superficial and deep cervical plexus block versus general anesthesia. The investigators did find a trend toward reduced risk of stroke and death, although this was at the cost of a slightly increased risk of MI. In patients with bilateral carotid disease, the composite outcome

Table 2
Complications of peripheral nerve blockade and how to minimize them

Complication	Strategy to Avoid
Infection	Hand washing, sterile preparation, cap, mask, and sterile gloves for single-shot blocks and full draping with sterile gowns for catheter placement
Hematoma	Minimize skin punctures, needle passes, optimize needle visualization
Local anesthetic toxicity/intravascular injection	Frequently aspiration during injection, limit total anesthetic dose
Nerve injury	Do not inject against pressure or if painful

of stroke, death, and MI was twice as frequent in patients under general anesthesia. In the analysis by Leichtle and colleagues,[8] preoperative neurologic dysfunction was associated with a significant increased rate of complications, notably MI, in patients undergoing CEA with general rather than regional anesthesia. At the least, there is a paucity of research showing inferiority with regional anesthesia as the primary anesthetic for CEA. Regional anesthesia is highly successful as the sole anesthetic technique for CEA, with conversion to general anesthesia reported in the range of 0% to 6%.[14,16–18]

Cutaneous innervation of the anterolateral neck originates as the ventral rami of cervical nerves C2, C3, and C4, which combine with C1 to form the deep cervical plexus. Four cutaneous nerves arise from the cervical plexus: the great auricular, lesser occipital, supraclavicular, and transverse cervical nerves. Regional blockade for CEA was historically accomplished with deep cervical plexus block, with or without a superficial cervical plexus block. However, several randomized, controlled trials have shown that a superficial cervical plexus block alone is as effective as when it is combined with a deep cervical plexus block with respect to operative conditions and patient satisfaction.[17,19–21] A systematic review by Pandit and colleagues[22] in 2007 showed that when a combined block is performed, the odds ratio of serious complications is 2.13 and of conversion to general anesthesia 5.15 compared with superficial cervical plexus block alone.

Because of confusion as to the depth of the superficial cervical plexus block, whether superficial or deep to the investing layer of fascia, a distinction in the nomenclature has been proposed. The superficial cervical plexus block is the subcutaneous injection occurring superficial to this investing fascia; the intermediate cervical plexus block is performed deep to the investing fascia but superficial to the deep cervical fascia. The intermediate cervical plexus mimics a deep cervical plexus block with fewer complications, taking advantage of the semipermeable nature of the deep cervical fascia, allowing spread of local anesthetic through the deep cervical fascia.[17] Although fewer side effects were observed with this block compared with the deep block, superiority of intermediate cervical plexus block to superficial cervical plexus block alone has not been established.[23,24]

Block supplementation by surgical injection of local anesthesia is frequently required with traditional approaches to cervical plexus blockade. Block failure or incomplete block is at least partially attributable to failure to provide anesthesia to the carotid sheath, which has contributions from the vagus nerve and the superior branch of ansa cervicalis.[18] Recently, Rossel and colleagues[25] described the technique of an intermediate cervical plexus block combined with ultrasound-guided perivascular injection, which reduced the rate of need of surgical injection to less than 20%. Ultrasound-guided perivascular injection was also used successfully by Martusevicius and colleagues,[18] but a head to head trial comparing these techniques with classic cervical plexus blocks has not been performed. In addition, ultrasound guidance has not been proved to be superior to landmark techniques for execution of the superficial cervical plexus block.[26]

Regional anesthesia can be accomplished with cervical epidural anesthesia; however, this is associated with increased incidence of hypotension, bradycardia, and bilateral phrenic nerve palsy, without improvement in analgesia or operating conditions.[27]

Cervical Plexus Blockade

Equipment

Sterile technique
1-cm to 5-cm short bevel needle

Local anesthetic, 15 to 25 mL
Optional: ultrasound guidance with a high-frequency linear probe

Patient preparation

The patient is positioned in the supine or semirecumbent position, with the head turned away from the site of surgery.

Technique best practices

Deep cervical plexus block

Landmark technique Nerve roots C1–C4 emerge from the gutters between the anterior and posterior tubercles of the tip of the corresponding transverse processes. The deep cervical plexus formed by C1–C4 is located immediately lateral to the tips of the transverse processes. The block can be performed as a single injection at the level of C4 or as multiple injections at C2, C3, and C4. There is no cutaneous contribution from nerve root C1. To perform the block, first draw a line connecting the mastoid process to the transverse process of C6, the latter being the most prominent transverse cervical process palpated just inferior to the cricoid cartilage and posterior to the clavicular head of the sternocleidomastoid muscle (SCM). Along this line, palpate or use ultrasonography to mark the transverse process of C2 located 1.5 to 2 cm caudad to the mastoid process, C3 3 to 4 cm, C4 4.5 to 6 cm. Clean the skin with antiseptic solution. Inject local anesthetic superficially along the entire marked line as the skin wheal. For each level, insert the needle perpendicular to the skin, with slight caudad and posterior orientation. Advance the needle slowly until contact is made with the transverse process, approximately 1 to 3 cm deep. Withdraw the needle 1 to 2 mm and inject 4 to 5 mL of local anesthetic in fractionated aliquots, while frequently aspirating for blood, because the vertebral artery typically is within 1 cm of the target. A single injection technique may alternatively be performed at the level of C4.[17,28,29] A total of 15 mL of local anesthetic as a single injection or spread over 3 levels is typically used.

Ultrasound guided To perform an ultrasound-guided block, a high-frequency linear probe can be positioned transversely at the level of the cricoid cartilage between the cricoid cartilage and SCM. From here, the probe is moved lateral to identify the prominent anterior tubercle characteristic of the C6 transverse process. Scanning cephalad, identify transverse processes and roots of C4, C3, and C2 and mark as sites of injection (**Fig. 1**).[30] Caudad tilt of the ultrasound probe may aid in identifying nerve roots. After cleansing skin and creating a skin wheal, the needle is advanced until

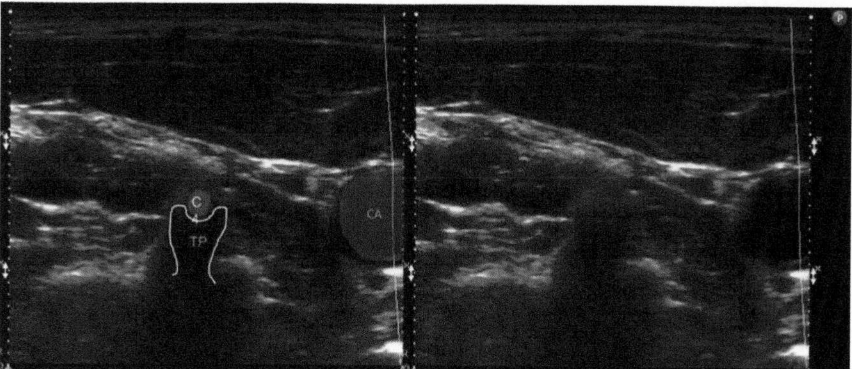

Fig. 1. Cervical nerve root 4 (C4) visualized between the anterior and posterior tubercle of the C4 transverse process (TP). The carotid artery (CA) is also visualized.

contact is made with the transverse process or the tip is seen close to the nerve root, and after negative aspiration, 5 mL local anesthetic is injected at each level.

Superficial cervical plexus block

Landmark technique The cutaneous branches of the cervical plexus converge just deep to the lateral border of the SCM, near the level of the cricoid cartilage. The superficial cervical plexus block is performed as a subcutaneous field block, with the needle inserted at this level. After cleaning with antiseptic solution and creating a skin wheal, the needle is inserted and guided just deep to the posterior border of the SCM (0.5 cm) and 5 mL of local anesthetic delivered. After this process, the needle is fanned superiorly and inferiorly; with each motion, an additional 5 mL of local anesthetic is delivered.[29]

Ultrasound guided To perform an ultrasound-guided block, place the ultrasound probe in transverse orientation at the midpoint of the posterior border of the SCM at approximately the level of the cricoid cartilage, visualizing the tapering edge of the SCM (**Fig. 2**). After cleaning the skin and producing a skin wheal, advance the needle from the posterior aspect just deep to the skin and platysma muscle until adjacent to the edge of the SCM. Five milliliters of local anesthetic is injected here after negative aspiration for blood. After initial injection, fan superiorly and inferiorly and inject as described earlier.

Intermediate cervical plexus block

Landmark technique The intermediate cervical plexus is performed by injecting local anesthetic just deep to the superficial cervical fascia. In identical fashion to the superficial cervical plexus block, the needle is inserted posterior to the SCM. The needle is advanced until a loss of resistance is felt, approximately 1 to 2 cm, and 15 to 25 mL of local anesthetic distributed in this space.[24]

Ultrasound guided To perform the ultrasound-guided block, place the ultrasound probe in transverse orientation at the midpoint of the posterior border of the SCM. The superficial cervical plexus may appear as a honeycomb orientation of hypoechoic structures at this level (see **Fig. 2**). If it is not visible, scan caudad or cephalad to identify the greater auricular nerve as it wraps around to the superficial aspect of the SCM. If the plexus is not visible, target the intermuscular plane deep to the tapering edge of

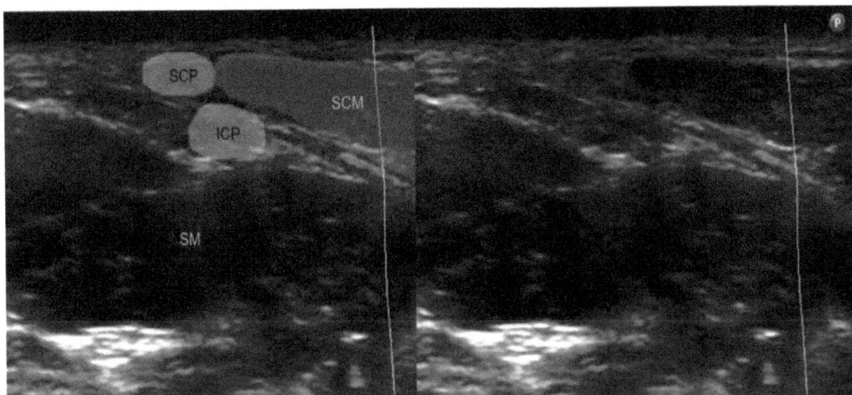

Fig. 2. The superficial cervical plexus (SCP) is visualized adjacent to the SCM. Deep to the superficial cervical fascia lies the intermediate cervical plexus (ICP). SM, anterior scalene muscle.

the SCM and superficial to the anterior and middle scalene muscles. Once the target is identified, clean the skin with antiseptic and create a skin wheal. The needle can be advanced until adjacent to the target. Ten to 15 mL of local anesthetic is injected in this location to complete the block.[29]

Perivascular injection

Position the ultrasound probe transversely just above the clavicle to identify the common carotid artery in cross section. Follow this cephalad to the bifurcation. After cleaning the skin and creating a skin wheal, advance the needle from the lateral border of the SCM until abutting the bifurcation point. After negative aspiration, local anesthetic is injected in this plane to achieve a half-moon shape spread.[18,25]

Postprocedure care

The onset time of the described blocks is approximately 10 to 20 minutes, depending on type, concentration, and volume of local anesthetic used. To test for adequate anesthesia, assess for loss of sensation to pinprick in the C2, C3, and C4 dermatome. Monitor the patient for signs of intrathecal, epidural, or intravascular injection, as well as phrenic nerve blockade, especially if a deep cervical plexus block is performed on patients with coexisting pulmonary disease. If regional anesthesia is performed for CEA at a center unfamiliar with its use, a discussion should be had with the surgical team about the expectation of requiring local supplementation, particularly to the carotid sheath.

Avoiding complications

The overall complication rate for all types of cervical plexus block is low. The composite of serious complications (including spinal anesthesia, respiratory distress, intravascular injection, and local anesthetic systemic toxicity) occurred in approximately 1% of patients receiving deep cervical blockade in a 2007 meta-analysis.[22] Virtually no serious block-related complications were reported in patients receiving a superficial cervical plexus block. A table of complications specific to cervical plexus blockade is provided (see **Table 2**).

OPEN REPAIR OF AAA

Open AAA repair has been performed in high-risk patients using combination spinal-epidural anesthesia without general anesthesia.[31,32] Although there has been success with this technique, neuraxial blockade is more commonly used in combination with a general anesthetic. Aside from superior analgesia, the benefits of this neuraxial analgesia for AAA versus intravenous pain control are controversial. Initial studies touted a reduction in postoperative hypertension[33] and time to extubation,[34] but absent were improvements in major cardiopulmonary morbidity or mortality. Although 1 group of investigators reported a 15% mortality reduction in patients with adjunctive epidural analgesia,[35] others have failed to replicate this finding. A 2012 meta-analysis found epidural superior to intravenous analgesia, with improved postoperative pain scores as well as a reduction in postoperative intubation times, acute respiratory failure rates, intensive care unit (ICU) stay duration, and rates of cardiac, gastrointestinal, and renal complications.[36] The counterpoint to these benefits is concern for postoperative coagulopathy, given large volume intraoperative blood loss and resuscitation, leading to increased risk of epidural hematoma.

Overall, the evidence for the use of adjunctive epidural analgesia for AAA repair is modest and must be weighed against the risk of postoperative coagulopathy for an individual patient. If an epidural is used, low thoracic, T8 to T10, is most appropriate.

The ideal anesthetic regimen is unclear, with some investigators[37] advocating use of epidural local anesthetic only after the aortic cross-clamp has been removed and hypotension resolved, or only postoperatively, or avoided all together in favor of epidural opioid alone.

An alternative adjunct to general anesthesia in patients at high risk for or refusing neuraxial blockade is the transversus abdominus plane (TAP) block. This block provides anesthesia only to the parietal peritoneum and abdominal wall, not to the viscera, and therefore cannot be used as the primary anesthetic.[28] Abdallah and colleagues[38] reported a case series of 6 patients undergoing open AAA with TAP blocks performed at the level of the iliac crest compared with their counterparts who refused TAP block. With a preoperative bilateral single-shot injection of 20 mL bupivacaine in the TAP, a 41.5% reduction in intraoperative opioid consumption, 42.2% reduction in us of postoperative morphine patient-controlled analgesia, decreased antiemetic requirements, and reduced pain scores for the first 48 hours were observed. Although the traditional approach to TAP blockade provides reliable analgesia only below the level of the umbilicus, a subcostal version is purported to extend this level to the upper abdomen. A study by Niraj and colleagues[39] compared subcostal TAP catheters versus epidural analgesia for upper abdominal surgery and found no difference in pain scores at 8 or 72 hours. Further research efforts are required to refine our knowledge of subcostal TAP block spread.

TAP Block

Sensation to the anterior abdominal wall is provided by ventral rami of T6-L1. In the lateral abdomen, these nerve roots lie in the fascial plane between transversus abdominus and internal oblique muscles, called the TAP.

Equipment

Sterile preparation
10-cm, 21-G needle
Local anesthetic, 20 to 30 mL per side
Ultrasound guidance with high-frequency linear probe

Patient preparation

This block can be performed with the patient either awake or asleep. The patient is positioned supine.

Technique best practices

A traditional TAP block is performed at the level of the iliac crest. The ultrasound probe is placed at this level in the midaxillary line, parallel to the muscles of the abdominal wall. The needle is advanced and guided deep to the fascia of the internal oblique just superficial to the transversus muscle (**Fig. 3**). Injection in this plane should create a clear fluid pocket dividing the 2 muscles. If the fluid pocket appears blurry, intramuscular injection should be suspected and the needle redirected slightly. To perform the subcostal block, simply complete these steps in the same plane just below the costal margin. A combination of blocks at both levels may be performed with care not to exceed safe doses of local anesthesia, because high plasma levels are expected after TAP block.[40] For either block, a perineural catheter may be threaded after localization of the needle in the TAP.

Postprocedure care

Postoperatively, the patient may be assessed for block success and visual analog pain scores. If a catheter was placed, the ideal regimen is unclear, with some advocating

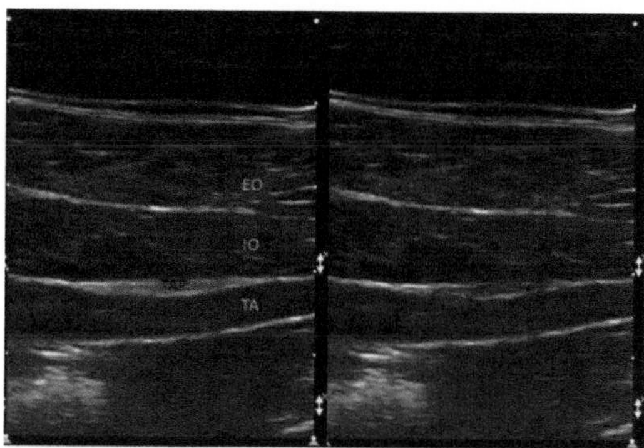

Fig. 3. TAP lies between the internal oblique (IO) and transversalis (TA) muscles, all deep to the external oblique (EO) muscle.

continuous infusion and others intermittent high-volume boluses. Confirmation of catheter injectate spread in the TAP can be performed under ultrasound guidance.

Avoiding complications

Although serious complications of TAP blocks, including liver lacerations and bowel perforation, have been reported, the overall complication rate is low, with most studies citing few to no adverse effects.[41]

ENDOVASCULAR REPAIR OF AAAS

Early endovascular repair of AAAs (EVAR) was performed solely under general anesthesia because of lengthy surgical duration and risk of open conversion. Procedure times and success rates have improved with experience, allowing for exploration of local and regional techniques as the primary anesthetic for EVAR.

Local anesthesia with intravenous sedation has been used with success across many centers,[42–46] primarily when femoral access is used for repair. Several investigators have reported decreased procedure times,[45–47] shorter ICU and hospital stays,[44,45,47–49] less vasopressor use,[43] and fewer cardiopulmonary complications[44,45,48–50] when local anesthesia is used in lieu of general anesthesia. Although theoretically at a disadvantage because of an inability to breath-hold during stent deployment, no difference in endoleak rate has been observed with local anesthesia.[47] Rates of conversion to general anesthesia have been reported as low as 0.5% of patients undergoing EVAR under local anesthesia.[44,45] However, local anesthesia is less feasible when complex dissection for iliac access is required.

Several regional anesthetic techniques have been used, including continuous spinal, epidural, combined spinal/epidural, paravertebral, and ilioinguinal/iliohypogastric blockade. However, most commonly, epidural or spinal has been used. A lack of reliable data exists for peripheral nerve blockade. Epidural or spinal anesthesia has been associated with decreased procedure duration,[43] length of ICU and hospital stay,[44,48] blood loss,[48] and pulmonary complications.[49] Adequate anesthesia is achieved for femoral or iliac approach with titration to a T10 level, often accomplished with blockade at the L3 to L4 or L4 to L5 level.

Although this evidence suggests a potential advantage for locoregional anesthesia compared with general anesthesia, the literature is largely retrospective. A recent meta-analysis by Karthikesalingam and colleagues[47] showed statistically significant improvements in postoperative complications, operative times, and hospital length of stay when general anesthesia is avoided. However, the investigators questioned the clinical relevance of the small absolute differences in the observed advantages. Although most studies have failed to show a mortality benefit with locoregional anesthesia, the EUROSTAR data analysis by Ruppert and colleagues[51] reported a reduction in mortality in the subset of ASA (American Society of Anesthesiologists) III–IV patients. Patients undergoing EVAR with locoregional anesthesia are typically sicker and are able to undergo aneurysm repair with similar mortality to healthier patients undergoing repair under general anesthesia.[44,47,48] However, complex aneurysms or difficult approaches to EVAR have commonly been cited as a reason for opting for general anesthesia.[47] Locoregional anesthesia may be of greatest benefit in high-risk patients undergoing relatively simple EVAR with femoral access.

LOWER EXTREMITY VASCULAR SURGERY: ARTERIAL BYPASS AND AMPUTATION

Regional anesthesia has been used for several decades for lower extremity vascular surgery. The proposed benefits of regional anesthetic techniques are improved hemodynamic stability, decreased catecholamine surge, and sympathectomy; all resulting in improved lower extremity blood flow.

For infrainguinal bypass surgery, hemodynamics may be better maintained with regional anesthesia, because heart rate volatility as well as the incidence of both intraoperative hypertension[52] and hypotension[53] have been shown to be more frequent with general anesthesia. Further, regional anesthesia is associated with decreased incidence of postoperative pneumonia.[54] Generally, however, tangible evidence of improvement in morbidity and mortality is sparse, and general anesthesia remains the technique of choice in more than 70% of procedures. This situation is surprising because, at the least, regional anesthesia is universally reported with at least equivalence of postoperative outcomes.[55–57] Therefore, epidural, spinal, and peripheral nerve blockade are acceptable anesthetic techniques for lower extremity vascular surgery.

A controversial point, but one in which regional anesthesia may have true benefit, is the effect of anesthetic technique on graft patency and return to the operating room. Multiple trials[54,58–60] have shown that general anesthesia is associated with increased likelihood of graft failure requiring regrafting, revision, or embolectomy. Others[57,61] have failed to replicate this result, and further prospective, randomized trials are required to verify this finding.

In the setting of lower extremity amputation, neuraxial anesthesia and peripheral nerve blockade have both been shown to significantly decrease perioperative pain.[62–65] A proposed additional benefit is a reduction in postoperative phantom limb pain, although this is not well supported by the literature with traditional perioperative management strategies. However, 1 promising observational study conducted by Borghi and colleagues[66] maintained sciatic and femoral perineural catheter infusions for a period of 4 to 83 days. Of patients compliant with the catheter protocol, 84% had zero pain at 1 year and only 39% had phantom limb phenomena, compared with the 60% to 70% of patients who experience phantom limb pain with traditional approaches.

Cutaneous innervation of the lower extremity is provided by the lumbar and lumbosacral plexi. The thigh is primarily innervated by the lumbar plexus, whereas the lumbosacral plexus provides innervation below the knee. The nerves of interest for most lower extremity bypass surgery are the femoral, a branch of the lumbar plexus, and sciatic, originating from the lumbosacral plexus. The lumbar plexus is composed of ventral rami from L1–L4, with a variable contribution from T12. The plexus itself is located deep to the psoas muscle adjacent to the transverse processes of lumbar vertebrae. The caudal portion of this plexus divides into the lateral femoral cutaneous, femoral, and obturator nerves responsible for leg innervation. The femoral nerve splits the iliopsoas muscle before coursing down the leg in the plane between the iliopsoas muscle and the fascia iliaca, just lateral to the femoral artery. The distribution of the femoral nerve includes sensory innervation to the anterior and medial thigh. The lumbosacral plexus is formed from ventral rami of L4-S3. From this plexus arises the sciatic nerve, which refers to the tibial and common peroneal nerves that course down the upper leg in a common sheath until they typically split at or near the popliteal fossa.[28]

The traditional means of providing regional anesthesia to the lower extremity is via epidural or intrathecal injection of local anesthetic. The involved dermatomes for bypass surgery are primarily L1–L4; a T10 level of anesthesia is achievable, with minimal hemodynamic compromise. A variety of local anesthetic solutions may be used for this purpose; discussion of these is beyond the scope of this article. Recently, performance of lower extremity bypass under peripheral nerve blockade was described. Yazigi and colleagues[67] provided a case series of 25 patients successfully undergoing infrainguinal bypass with combination femoral and sciatic nerve blockade, supplemented by intravenous midazolam. Astounding hemodynamic stability was observed in these patients, with only 2 requiring vasopressor support, and zero patients required conversion to general anesthesia. The investigators followed with a prospective, randomized study[68] comparing this technique with general anesthesia for infrainguinal bypass, which showed a statistically significant reduction in intraoperative myocardial ischemia, as defined by 1 minute or greater ST segment changes, in the group randomized to peripheral nerve blockade. Other approaches have included combined femoral, sciatic, and obturator blockade or combined psoas, sciatic, and T12-L1 paravertebral blockade.[69] Ultrasound-guided approaches to the femoral and sciatic nerve blocks are discussed here.

Femoral Nerve Blockade

Equipment

- Sterile technique
- 10-cm block needle
- 20 mL of local anesthetic
- Ultrasound guidance with a high-frequency linear probe

Patient preparation

The patient is positioned supine.

Technique best practices

Place the ultrasound probe in the inguinal crease, near the midline of the thigh. Identify the pulsatile femoral artery; the nerve lies laterally to this structure. The nerve should appear as a hyperechoic bundle at this level. The fascia iliaca appears as a thin hyperechoic strip superficial to the nerve and extending medial and deep to the artery (**Fig. 4**). Once the fascia iliaca is identified, the skin is prepared and a skin wheal made. The needle is advanced just deep to the fascia iliaca. Local anesthetic injected in this plane should be visualized coursing above or below the nerve and deep to the femoral artery. A catheter can be threaded to provide continuous analgesia.

Postprocedure care

Success of the block can be confirmed by assessing loss of sensation to pinprick over the anterior thigh and medial calf, as well as by assessing quadriceps femoris

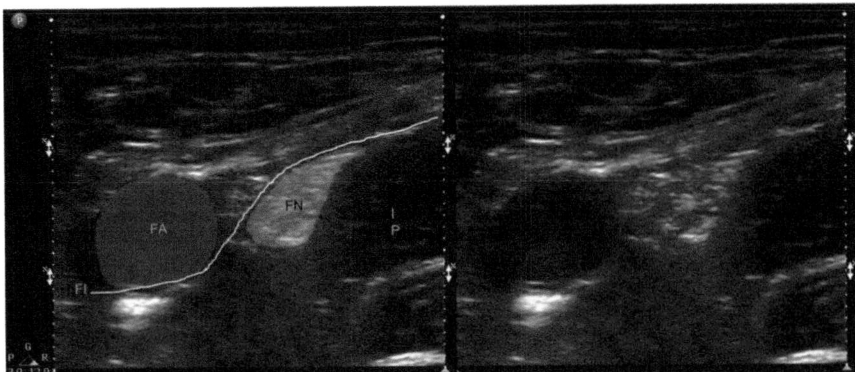

Fig. 4. The femoral nerve (FN) lies immediately lateral to the femoral artery (FA). The 2 are divided by the fascia iliaca (FI), leading to the characteristic spread of local anesthetic from the nerve under the artery. The iliopsoas muscle (IP) is also visualized.

weakness. The catheter should be secured with adhesive dressing. For postoperative pain management, an infusion of bupivacaine 0.125% or ropivacaine 0.2% is appropriate.

Avoiding complications

A 5.7% vascular puncture risk has been reported,[70] avoided best with optimal needle imaging and frequent aspiration. Weakness of the quadriceps muscle is expected, and fall precautions should be closely observed while this block is in place.

Sciatic Nerve Blockade

Several approaches (anterior, parasacral, transgluteal, and subgluteal) are available for ultrasound-guided proximal sciatic nerve blockade. Because the anterior approach is deep and less suitable for catheter techniques, and the parasacral approach without specific benefit, only the subgluteal and infragluteal approaches are described here.

Equipment

Sterile technique
10-cm block needle
20 to 30 mL of local anesthetic
Ultrasound guidance with a linear or curvilinear probe, depending on body habitus

Positioning

The patient may be positioned lateral, prone, or supine with leg elevated.

Technique best practices

The sciatic nerve can be blocked anywhere along its path as it courses down the leg. More proximal approaches are preferred to adequately cover the surgical site. Start the scan by placing the transducer transversely at the infragluteal crease. The sciatic nerve is then identified as an elliptical hyperechoic structure between the greater trochanter and ischial tuberosity under the gluteus maximus at the subgluteal level (**Fig. 5**). The nerve is found deep to the biceps femoris for more distal approaches. After sterile preparation and skin wheal formation, the needle is advanced toward the edge of the sciatic nerve. Injection around the sciatic nerve produces a circumferential pattern of local anesthetic. A catheter can be threaded to provide prolonged analgesia and sympathectomy.

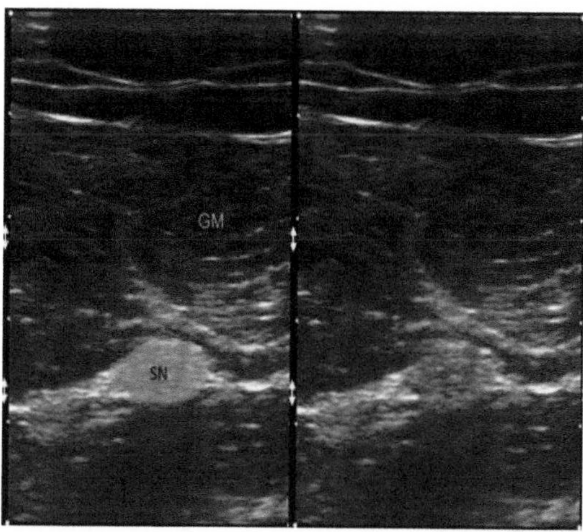

Fig. 5. The sciatic nerve (SN) appears as a hyperechoic bundle just deep to the gluteus muscle (GM).

Postprocedure care

Success of the block can be confirmed by assessing loss of sensation to pinprick on the posterior and lateral aspects of the calf. The catheter should be secured with adhesive dressing. For postoperative pain management, an infusion of bupivacaine 0.125% or ropivacaine 0.2% is appropriate.

Avoiding complications

Intraneural injection may be relatively common in sciatic nerve blockade, reported by Hara and colleagues[71] as occurring in 16% of patients, avoided by optimizing visualization of the needle tip and injecting with low pressure. Sciatic blockade is also associated with a 6.3% vascular puncture risk.[70]

AVF CREATION

A persistent problem with AVF creation is the approximate 25% failure rate.[72] Two important predictors for success of AVF maturation are vein diameter and blood flow.[72] Peripheral nerve blockade creates a sympathectomy, resulting in vasodilation, increased fistula blood flow, and perhaps decreased failure rate. Venodilation with regional anesthesia has been reported in numerous studies,[72–76] with percent dilation ranging from 8.7% to 35%. This vasodilation has been shown to improve site selection[77] and allow fistula creation in patients otherwise scheduled for arteriovenous grafting. Sahin and colleagues[78] performed a randomized, prospective trial comparing local infiltration with infraclavicular blockade for AVF surgery. Fistula flow was statistically significantly greater at 3 hours, 7 days, and 8 weeks after surgery in the infraclavicular patient group. Elsharawy and Al-metwalli,[79] alternatively, were unable to show a difference in graft failure rate comparing general anesthesia with brachial plexus block. Overall, a retrospective review article[72] from 2009 reported reduced vasospasm, shorter fistula maturation times, lower failure rates, and higher patency rates with regional blockade. Further, regional anesthesia has been associated with decreased anesthesia dedicated time for ambulatory upper extremity surgery.[80]

Brachial plexus block can be performed at a variety of levels to provide adequate anesthesia for AVF creation. Most cutaneous sensation to the surgical field for distal fistula creation is provided by the musculocutaneous and medial antebrachial cutaneous nerves. These 2 nerves were selectively anesthetized in case series,[81,82] providing adequate anesthesia for 75% and 83% of patients. The remaining required surgical supplementation when the surgical field drifted into radial nerve territory.

Most investigators perform nonselective brachial plexus block. The surgical field may include radial, axillary, and intercostobrachial nerve territory; the latter of which is not consistently blocked with all brachial plexus block approaches. Niemi and colleagues[83] compared axillary and infraclavicular brachial plexus blocks for AVF creation without significant difference in outcomes, although musculocutaneous blockade set in faster with infraclavicular block. Any approach (supraclavicular, infraclavicular, or axillary) to brachial plexus blockade is appropriate for AVF creation. A comparison of ultrasound-guided approaches to each block performed by Tran and colleagues[84] reported no differences in success rates or serious complication rates. Single and double injection techniques generate similar success with infraclavicular and supraclavicular blockade, whereas a double injection approach is adequate for axillary blockade. Supraclavicular or infraclavicular approaches are preferred to minimize needle passes in this population likely to receive anticoagulation. Overall, ultrasound-guided approaches are superior to blind or nerve-stimulating approaches.[85–87] A single-shot approach is generally adequate for this procedure. If the procedure is performed with a primary anesthetic, a surgical concentration of local anesthetic should be chosen. To block the medial skin of the upper arm for proximal AVF surgery, the infraclavicular block may be sufficient or may be supplemented by the intercostobrachial block.

Supraclavicular Nerve Blockade

Equipment

Sterile technique
5-cm to 10-cm 21-G block needle
20 to 30 mL of local anesthetic
Ultrasound guidance with a high-frequency linear probe

Patient preparation

Patient supine or semirecumbent, head turned away.

Technique best practices

Place the transducer parallel to the clavicle in the supraclavicular fossa. The subclavian artery should be identified in cross section, with the brachial plexus trunks seen as hypoechoic structures surrounding the artery laterally or superiorly (**Fig. 6**). The first rib is visualized as the hyperechoic line at the inferior margin of the artery. Apply color

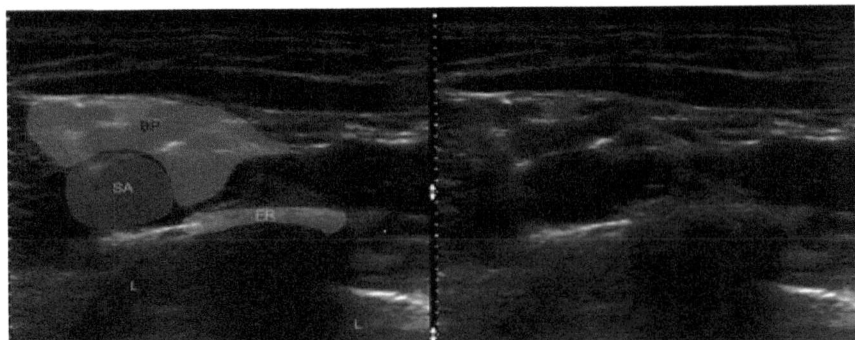

Fig. 6. Brachial plexus (BP) distribution surrounding the subclavian artery (SA). Note the proximity to the first rib (FR) and lung (L).

to assess the vessels that traverse the plexus. After sterile preparation and skin wheal formation, the needle is directed to the inferolateral edge of the subclavian artery, the corner pocket.[88] After negative aspiration, 20 mL of local anesthetic is injected. Sometimes, the plexus is separated by a fascial layer or vessel that prevents complete spread of the solution,[89] in which case, the needle should be redirected and solution injected to ensure that all parts of the plexus are exposed to local anesthetic.

Postprocedure care
Onset of the block can be confirmed early by assessing for vasodilation and relative warmth of the blocked limb. Loss of sensation to pinprick in the musculocutaneous and medial antebrachial nerve distribution as well as motor blockade confirms the onset of surgical anesthesia.

Infraclavicular Nerve Blockade

Equipment

Sterile technique
5-cm to 10-cm 21-G block needle
20 to 30 mL of local anesthetic
Ultrasound guidance with a high-frequency linear probe

Patient preparation
Patient supine or semirecumbent, head turned away, arm abducted 90° to displace clavicle.

Technique best practices
Place the transducer inferior to the clavicle, just medial to the coracoid process. Identify the pulsating subclavian artery. Rotate and adjust the angle of the probe to optimize the cross-sectional view of the vessel. Here, the lateral, posterior, and medial cords of the brachial plexus are visible surrounding the artery (**Fig. 7**). After sterile preparation and skin wheal formation, advance the needle toward the posterior aspect of the neurovascular bundle. A single injection posterior to the artery is adequate, unless initial spread does not create a reassuring U shape around the artery, in which case, the needle must be redirected and additional injection performed to account for this.

Postprocedure care
Onset of the block can be confirmed early by assessing for vasodilation and relative warmth of the blocked limb. Loss of sensation to pinprick in the musculocutaneous and medial antebrachial nerve distribution and motor blockade confirm the onset of surgical anesthesia.

Avoiding complications
Compared with supraclavicular blockade, the risk of phrenic nerve block or Horner syndrome is negligible.

Intercostobrachial Blockade

Equipment

Sterile preparation
5-cm to 10-cm block needle
10 mL of local anesthetic

Patient preparation
Patient supine, arm abducted 90°.

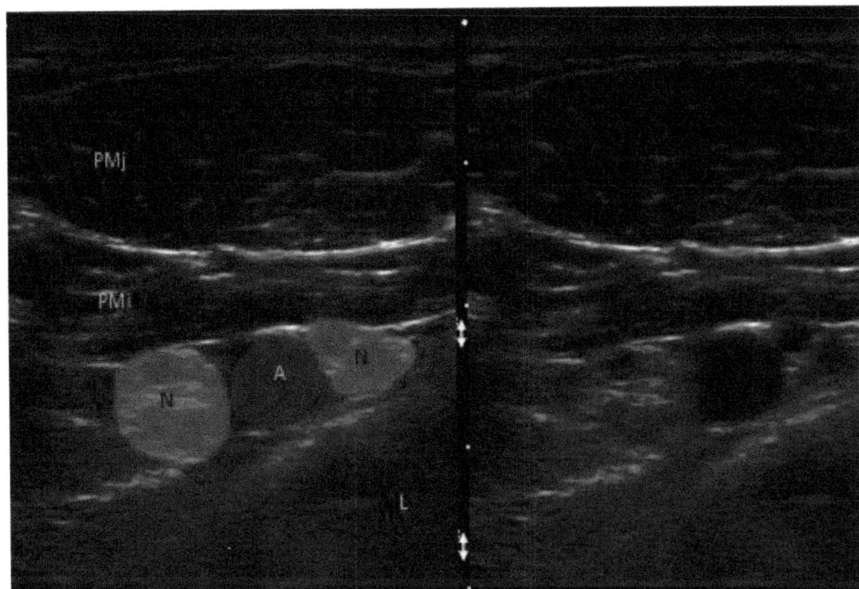

Fig. 7. Infraclavicular nerve block. Deep to pectoralis major (PMj) and minor (PMi) lies the brachial plexus (N) surrounding the axillary artery (A). The medial and lateral cords are clearly shown, whereas the posterior cord, deep to the artery, may be difficult to appreciate. Note the proximity to the lung (L).

Technique best practices

This block is performed as a subcutaneous field block within the axilla. After sterile preparation, the needle is inserted at the proximal aspect of the axilla and advanced subcutaneously to the inferior aspect. Local anesthetic is injected continuously as the needle is removed to form a linear skin wheal.

Postprocedure care

The onset of the intercostobrachial block is rapid and can be assessed by testing loss of sensation to pinprick over the medial upper arm.

Avoiding complications

No block-specific complications. Generalized complications of peripheral nerve blockade are avoided by remaining within the subcutaneous layer during needle advancement.

SUMMARY

Regional anesthesia is an acceptable modality to be used as the primary anesthetic technique or as an adjunct to general anesthesia for vascular surgery. When performed by the experienced anesthesiologist, these techniques may improve morbidity and analgesia and reduce hospital stays in this challenging patient population. Overall, however, data from randomized, controlled trials are lacking, and therefore, general anesthesia remains an appropriate alternative. The decision to use regional techniques should be made by the patient, surgeon, and anesthesiologist after an individualized discussion of the risk benefit profile for each patient and surgery.

REFERENCES

1. Feringa HH, Karagiannis SE, Vidakovic R, et al. The prevalence and prognosis of unrecognized myocardial infarction and silent myocardial ischemia in patients undergoing major vascular surgery. Coron Artery Dis 2007;18(7):571–6.
2. Musallam KM, Rosendaal FR, Zaatari G, et al. Smoking and the risk of mortality and vascular and respiratory events in patients undergoing major surgery. JAMA Surg 2013;148(8):755–62.
3. Horlocker TT, Wedel DJ, Rowlingson JC, et al. Regional anesthesia in the patient receiving antithrombotic or thrombolytic therapy: American Society of Regional Anesthesia and Pain Medicine Evidence-Based Guidelines. Reg Anesth Pain Med 2010;35(1):64–101.
4. Rockman CB, Riles TS, Gold M, et al. A comparison of regional and general anesthesia in patients undergoing carotid endarterectomy. J Vasc Surg 1996; 24:946–56.
5. Corson JD, Chang BB, Shah DM, et al. The influence of anesthetic choice on carotid endarterectomy outcome. Arch Surg 1987;122(7):807–12.
6. Lutz HJ, Michael R, Gahl B, et al. Local versus general anaesthesia for carotid endarterectomy–improving the gold standard? Eur J Vasc Endovasc Surg 2008; 36:145–9.
7. Mracek J, Holeckova I, Chytra I, et al. The impact of general versus local anesthesia on early subclinical cognitive function following carotid endarterectomy evaluated using P3 event-related potentials. Acta Neurochir 2012;154: 433–8.
8. Leichtle SW, Mouawad NJ, Welch K, et al. Outcomes of carotid endarterectomy under general and regional anesthesia from the American College of Surgeons' National Surgical Quality Improvement Program. J Vasc Surg 2012;56:81–8.
9. Becquemin JP, Paris E, Valverde A, et al. Carotid surgery. Is regional anesthesia always appropriate? J Cardiovasc Surg (Torino) 1991;32(5):592–8.
10. Sternbach Y, Illig KA, Zhang R, et al. Hemodynamic benefits of regional anesthesia for carotid endarterectomy. J Vasc Surg 2002;35:333–9.
11. Watts K, Lin PH, Bush RL. The impact of anesthetic modality on the outcome of carotid endarterectomy. Am J Surg 2004;188:741–7.
12. Lewis SC, Warlow CP, Bodenham AR, et al. General anaesthesia versus local anaesthesia for carotid surgery (GALA): a multicentre, randomised controlled trial. Lancet 2008;372:2132–42.
13. Messner M, Albrecht S, Lang W, et al. The superficial cervical plexus block for postoperative pain therapy in carotid artery surgery. A prospective randomised controlled trial. Eur J Vasc Endovasc Surg 2007;33:50–4.
14. Markovic D, Vlajkovic G, Sindjelic R, et al. Cervical plexus block versus general anesthesia in carotid surgery: single center experience. Arch Med Sci 2012; 8(6):1035–40.
15. Guay J. Regional or general anesthesia for carotid endarterectomy? Evidence from published prospective and retrospective studies. J Cardiothorac Vasc Anesth 2007;21(1):127–32.
16. Hariharan S, Naraynsingh V, Esack A, et al. Perioperative outcome of carotid endarterectomy with regional anesthesia: two decades of experience from the Caribbean. J Clin Anesth 2010;22:169–73.
17. Pandit JJ, Bree S, Dillon P, et al. A comparison of superficial versus combined (superficial and deep) cervical plexus block for carotid endarterectomy: a prospective, randomized study. Anesth Analg 2000;91:781–6.

18. Martusevicius R, Swiatek F, Joergensen LG, et al. Ultrasound-guided locoregional anaesthesia for carotid endarterectomy: a prospective observational study. Eur J Vasc Endovasc Surg 2012;44:27–30.
19. Stoneham MD, Doyle AR, Knighton JD, et al. Prospective, randomized comparison of deep or superficial cervical plexus block for carotid endarterectomy surgery. Anesthesiology 1998;89:907–12.
20. de Sousa AA, Filho MA, Faglione W, et al. Superficial vs combined cervical plexus block for carotid endarterectomy: a prospective, randomized study. Surg Neurol 2005;63:22–5.
21. Ivanec Z, Mazul-Sunkol B, Lovricevic I, et al. Superficial versus combined (deep and superficial) cervical plexus block for carotid endarterectomy. Acta Clin Croat 2008;47(2):81–6.
22. Pandit JJ, Satya-Krishna R, Gration P. Superficial or deep cervical plexus block for carotid endarterectomy: a systematic review of complications. Br J Anaesth 2007;99(2):159–69.
23. Barone M, Diemunsch P, Baldassarre E, et al. Carotid endarterectomy with intermediate cervical plexus block. Tex Heart Inst J 2010;37(3):297–300.
24. Ramachandran SK, Picton P, Shanks A, et al. Comparison of intermediate vs subcutaneous cervical plexus block for carotid endarterectomy. Br J Anaesth 2011;107(2):157–63.
25. Rossel T, Kersting S, Heller A, et al. Combination of high-resolution ultrasound-guided perivascular regional anesthesia of the internal carotid artery and intermediate cervical plexus block for carotid surgery. Ultrasound Med Biol 2013;39(6):981–6.
26. Tran DQ, Dugani S, Finlayson R. A randomized comparison between ultrasound-guided and landmark-based superficial cervical plexus block. Reg Anesth Pain Med 2010;35:539–43.
27. Hakl M, Michalek P, Sevcik P, et al. Regional anaesthesia for carotid endarterectomy: an audit over 10 years. Br J Anaesth 2007;99(3):415–20.
28. Brown DL. Atlas of regional anesthesia. Philadelphia: Saunders; 2010.
29. Gray AT. Atlas of ultrasound-guided regional anesthesia. Philadelphia: Saunders; 2013.
30. Soeding P, Eizenberg N. Review article: anatomical considerations for ultrasound guidance for regional anesthesia of the neck and upper limb. Can J Anaesth 2009;6:518–33.
31. Berardi G, Ferrero E, Fadde M, et al. Combined spinal and epidural anesthesia for open abdominal aortic aneurysm surgery in vigil patients with severe chronic obstructive pulmonary disease ineligible for endovascular aneurysm repair. Analysis of results and description of technique. Int Angiol 2010;29(3):278–83.
32. Flores JA, Nishibe T, Koyama M, et al. Combined spinal and epidural anesthesia for abdominal aortic aneurysm surgery in patients with severe chronic obstructive pulmonary disease. Int Angiol 2002;21(3):218–21.
33. Breslow MJ, Jordan DA, Christopherson R, et al. Epidural morphine decreases postoperative hypertension by attenuating sympathetic nervous system hyperactivity. JAMA 1989;261:3577–81.
34. Norris EJ, Beattie C, Perler BA, et al. Double-masked randomized trial comparing alternate combinations of intraoperative anesthesia and postoperative analgesia in abdominal aortic surgery. Anesthesiology 2001;95:1054–67.
35. Park WY, Thompson JS, Lee KK, et al. Effect of epidural anesthesia and analgesia on perioperative outcome. Ann Surg 2001;234(4):560–71.

36. Nishimori M, Low JH, Zheng H, et al. Epidural pain relief versus systemic opioid-based pain relief for abdominal aortic surgery. Cochrane Database Syst Rev 2012;(7):CD005059.
37. Miller R, Erikkson LI, Fleisher LA, et al. Miller's anesthesia. 7th edition. Philadelphia: Churchill Livingstone; 2010.
38. Abdallah FW, Adham AM, Chan VW, et al. Analgesic benefits of preincisional transversus abdominis plane block for abdominal aortic aneurysm repair. J Cardiothorac Vasc Anesth 2013;27(3):536–8.
39. Niraj G, Kelkar A, Jeyapalan I, et al. Comparison of analgesic efficacy of subcostal transversus abdominis plane blocks with epidural analgesia following upper abdominal surgery. Anaesthesia 2011;66:465–71.
40. Griffiths JD, Barron FA, Grant S, et al. Plasma ropivacaine concentrations after ultrasound-guided transversus abdominis plane block. Br J Anaesth 2010; 105(6):853–6.
41. Charlton S, Cyna AM, Middleton P, et al. Perioperative transversus abdominis plane (TAP) blocks for analgesia after abdominal surgery. Cochrane Database Syst Rev 2010;(12):CD007705.
42. Virgilio C, Romero L, Donayre C, et al. Endovascular abdominal aortic aneurysm repair with general versus local anesthesia: a comparison of cardiopulmonary morbidity and mortality rates. J Vasc Surg 2002;36:988–91.
43. Bettex DA, Lachat M, Pfammatter T, et al. To compare general, epidural, and local anaesthesia for endovascular aneurysm repair. Eur J Vasc Endovasc Surg 2001;21:179–84.
44. Ruppert V, Leurs LJ, Steckmeier B, et al. Influence of anesthesia type on outcome after endovascular aortic aneurysm repair: an analysis based on EUROSTAR data. J Vasc Surg 2006;44:16–21.
45. Verhoeven EL, Cina CS, Tielliu IF, et al. Local anesthesia for endovascular abdominal aortic aneurysm repair. J Vasc Surg 2005;42:402–9.
46. Asakura Y, Ishibashi H, Ishiguchi T, et al. General versus locoregional anesthesia for endovascular aortic aneurysm repair: influences of the type of anesthesia on its outcome. J Anesth 2009;23:158–61.
47. Karthikesalingam A, Thrumurthy SG, Young EL, et al. Locoregional anesthesia for endovascular aneurysm repair. J Vasc Surg 2012;56:510–9.
48. Parra JR, Crabtree T, McLafferty RB, et al. Anesthesia technique and outcomes of endovascular aneurysm repair. Ann Vasc Surg 2005;19:123–9.
49. Edwards MS, Andrews JS, Edwards AF, et al. Results of endovascular aortic aneurysm repair with general, regional, and local/monitored anesthesia care in the American College of Surgeons National Surgical Quality Improvement Program database. J Vasc Surg 2011;54:1273–82.
50. Bakker EJ, van de Luijtgaarden KM, van Lier F, et al. General anaesthesia is associated with adverse cardiac outcome after endovascular aneurysm repair. Eur J Vasc Endovasc Surg 2012;44:121–5.
51. Ruppert V, Leurs LJ, Rieger J, et al. Risk-adapted outcome after endovascular aortic aneurysm repair: analysis of anesthesia types based on EUROSTAR data. J Endovasc Ther 2007;14:12–22.
52. Christopherson R, Glavan NJ, Norris EJ, et al. Control of blood pressure and heart rate in patients randomized to epidural or general anesthesia for lower extremity vascular surgery. J Clin Anesth 1996;8:578–84.
53. Damask MC, Weissman C, Todd G. General versus epidural anesthesia for femoral-popliteal bypass surgery. J Clin Anesth 1990;2:71–5.

54. Singh N, Sidawy AN, Dezee K, et al. The effects of the type of anesthesia on outcomes of lower extremity infrainguinal bypass. J Vasc Surg 2006;44(5):964–70.
55. Bode RH, Lewis KP, Zarich SW, et al. Cardiac outcome after peripheral vascular surgery. Comparison of general and regional anesthesia. Anesthesiology 1996; 84:3–13.
56. Rivers SP, Scher LA, Sheehan E, et al. Epidural versus general anesthesia for infrainguinal arterial reconstruction. J Vasc Surg 1991;14(6):764–8.
57. Barbosa FT, Juca MJ, Castro AA, et al. Neuraxial anaesthesia for lower-limb revascularization. Cochrane Database Syst Rev 2013;(7):CD007083.
58. Perler BA, Christopherson R, Rosenfeld BA, et al. The influence of anesthetic method on infrainguinal bypass graft patency: a closer look. Am Surg 1995; 61(9):784–9.
59. Christopherson R, Beattie C, Frank SM, et al. Perioperative morbidity in patients randomized to epidural or general anesthesia for lower extremity vascular surgery. Anesthesiology 1993;79(3):422–34.
60. Ghanami RJ, Hurie J, Andrews JS, et al. Anesthesia-based evaluation of outcomes of lower-extremity vascular bypass procedures. Ann Vasc Surg 2013; 27:199–207.
61. Pierce ET, Pomposelli FB, Stanley GD, et al. Anesthesia type does not influence early graft patency or limb salvage rates of lower extremity arterial bypass. J Vasc Surg 1997;25:226–33.
62. Ong BY, Arneja A, Ong EW. Effects of anesthesia on pain after lower-limb amputation. J Clin Anesth 2006;18:600–4.
63. Sahin SH, Colak A, Arar C, et al. A retrospective trial comparing the effects of different anesthetic techniques on phantom pain after lower limb amputation. Curr Ther Res Clin Exp 2011;72:127–37.
64. Becotte A, de Medicis E, Lapie V, et al. Preoperative continuous sciatic nerve block for perioperative analgesia and for phantom limb pain. J Clin Anesth 2012;24(3):256–7.
65. Karanikolas M, Aretha D, Tsolakis I, et al. Optimized perioperative analgesia reduces chronic phantom limb pain intensity, prevalence, and frequency. Anesthesiology 2011;111(5):1144–54.
66. Borghi B, D'Addabbo M, White PF, et al. The use of prolonged peripheral neural blockade after lower extremity amputation: the effect on symptoms associated with phantom limb syndrome. Anesth Analg 2010;111:1308–15.
67. Yazigi A, Madi-Gebara S, Haddad F, et al. Combined sciatic and femoral nerve blocks for infrainguinal arterial bypass surgery: a case series. J Cardiothorac Vasc Anesth 2005;19(2):220–1.
68. Yazigi A, Madi-Gebara S, Haddad F, et al. Intraoperative myocardial ischemia in peripheral vascular surgery: general anesthesia vs combined sciatic and femoral nerve blocks. J Clin Anesth 2005;17:499–503.
69. Basagan-Mogol E, Turker G, Yilmaz M, et al. Combination of a psoas compartment, sciatic nerve, and T12-L1 paravertebral blocks for femoropopliteal bypass surgery in a high-risk patient. J Cardiothorac Vasc Anesth 2008;22(2):337–9.
70. Jeng CL, Torrillo TM, Rosenblatt MA. Complications of peripheral nerve blocks. Br J Anaesth 2010;105:97–107.
71. Hara K, Sakura S, Yokokawa N, et al. Incidence and effects of unintentional intraneural injection during ultrasound-guided subgluteal sciatic nerve block. Reg Anesth Pain Med 2012;37(3):289–93.
72. Malinzak EB, Gan TJ. Regional anesthesia for vascular access surgery. Anesth Analg 2009;109:976–80.

73. Hingorani AP, Ascher E, Gupta P, et al. Regional anesthesia: preferred technique for venodilatation in the creation of upper extremity arteriovenous fistulae. Vascular 2006;14(1):23–6.
74. Reynolds TS, Kim KM, Dukkipati R, et al. Pre-operative regional block anesthesia enhances operative strategy for arteriovenous fistula creation. J Vasc Access 2011;12(4):336–40.
75. Lo Monte A, Damiano G, Mularo A, et al. Comparison between local and regional anesthesia in arteriovenous fistula creation. J Vasc Access 2011;12(4):331–5.
76. Shemesh D, Olsha O, Orkin D, et al. Sympathectomy-like effects of brachial plexus block in arteriovenous access surgery. Ultrasound Med Biol 2006;32(6):817–22.
77. Laskowski IA, Muhs B, Rockman CR, et al. Regional nerve block allows for optimization of planning in the creation of arteriovenous access for hemodialysis by improving superficial venous dilatation. Ann Vasc Surg 2007;21:730–3.
78. Sahin L, Gul R, Mizrak A, et al. Ultrasound-guided infraclavicular brachial plexus block enhances postoperative blood flow in arteriovenous fistulas. J Vasc Surg 2011;54:749–53.
79. Elsharawy MA, Al-metwalli R. Does regional anesthesia influence early outcome of upper arm arteriovenous fistula? Saudi J Kidney Dis Transpl 2010;21(6):1048–52.
80. Mariano ER, Chu LF, Peinado CR, et al. Anesthesia-controlled time and turnover time for ambulatory upper extremity surgery performed with regional versus general anesthesia. J Clin Anesth 2009;21(4):253–7.
81. Eldredge SJ, Sperry RJ, Johnson JO. Regional anesthesia for arteriovenous fistula creation in the forearm: a new approach. Anesthesiology 1992;77:1230–1.
82. Viscomi CM, Reese J, Rathmell JP. Medial and lateral antebrachial cutaneous nerve blocks: an easily learned regional anesthetic for forearm arteriovenous fistula surgery. Reg Anesth 1996;21(1):2–5.
83. Niemi TT, Salmela L, Aromaa U, et al. Single-injection brachial plexus anesthesia for arteriovenous fistula surgery of the forearm: a comparison of infraclavicular coracoid and axillary approach. Reg Anesth Pain Med 2007;32(1):55–9.
84. Tran DQ, Russo G, Munoz L, et al. A prospective, randomized comparison between ultrasound-guided supraclavicular, infraclavicular, and axillary brachial plexus blocks. Reg Anesth Pain Med 2009;34:366–71.
85. Tran DQ, Bertini P, Zaouter C, et al. A prospective, randomized comparison between single- and double-injection ultrasound-guided infraclavicular brachial plexus block. Reg Anesth Pain Med 2010;35:16–21.
86. Tran DQ, Munoz L, Zaouter C, et al. A prospective, randomized comparison between single- and double-injection, ultrasound-guided supraclavicular brachial plexus block. Reg Anesth Pain Med 2009;34:420–4.
87. Tran DQ, Pham K, Dugani S, et al. A prospective, randomized comparison between double-, triple-, and quadruple-injection ultrasound-guided axillary brachial plexus block. Reg Anesth Pain Med 2012;37:248–53.
88. Soares LG, Brull R, Lai J, et al. Eight ball, corner pocket: the optimal needle position for ultrasound-guided supraclavicular block. Reg Anesth Pain Med 2007;32:94–5.
89. Abrahams MS, Aziz MF, Fu RF, et al. Ultrasound guidance compared with electrical neurostimulation for peripheral nerve block: a systematic review and meta-analysis of randomized controlled trials. Br J Anaesth 2009;102:408–17.

Perioperative Management of Lower Extremity Revascularization

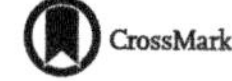

James M. Anton, MD[a,b,*], Marie LaPenta McHenry, MD[c]

KEYWORDS

• Peripheral arterial disease • Atherosclerosis • Revascularization of lower extremity • Neuraxial blockade • General anesthesia • Cardiovascular morbidity • Graft patency

KEY POINTS

- Patients presenting for lower extremity revascularization often have multiple systemic comorbidities, making them high-risk surgical candidates.
- Neuraxial anesthesia and general anesthesia are equivocal in their effect on perioperative cardiac morbidity and improved graft patency.
- Postoperative epidural analgesia may improve perioperative cardiac morbidity.
- Systemic antithrombotic and anticoagulation therapy is common among this patient population and may affect anesthetic techniques.

INTRODUCTION

Peripheral arterial disease (PAD) is a disease with significant morbidity and mortality. The recent focus on early screening and detection, aggressive medical management, and modification of risk factors has allowed many patients to avoid or delay more aggressive surgical intervention. The consequence of these practices is that a large majority of patients presenting for surgical lower extremity revascularization, through either endovascular or open techniques, have advanced systemic atherosclerotic disease involving not only peripheral limbs but also coronary, cerebral, and renal circulations. Vascular patients are among those with the highest perioperative risk, making them a challenge even for experienced anesthesiologists. Appropriate management of these patients requires an understanding of the pathophysiology of the disease, common comorbidities, perioperative complications, and possible surgical intervention strategies.

[a] St. Luke's Medical Group, CHI St. Luke's Health, 6720 Bertner Avenue, Room 0520, MC 1-226, Houston, TX 77030, USA; [b] Division of Cardiovascular Anesthesiology, Texas Heart Institute, Baylor St. Luke's Medical Center, 6720 Bertner Avenue, Room 0520, MC 1-226, Houston, TX 77030, USA; [c] Department of Anesthesiology, Perioperative and Pain Medicine, Stanford Hospital and Clinics, 300 Pasteur Drive, Stanford, CA 94305, USA
* Corresponding author. Division of Cardiovascular Anesthesiology, Texas Heart Institute, Baylor St. Luke's Medical Center, 6720 Bertner Avenue, Room 0520, MC 1-226, Houston, TX 77030.
E-mail address: james.anton@sbcglobal.net

Anesthesiology Clin 32 (2014) 661–676
http://dx.doi.org/10.1016/j.anclin.2014.05.004 anesthesiology.theclinics.com
1932-2275/14/$ – see front matter

PERIPHERAL ARTERIAL DISEASE

Epidemiology

PAD is common, affecting 3% to 10% of people younger than 70 years and 15% to 20% of people over age 70.[1] Globally, the number of people with PAD has increased by nearly one-fourth between 2000 and 2010,[2] despite the understanding that treatment of modifiable risk factors may decrease the burden of this disease. Lower limb PAD, specifically, is the third leading cause of atherosclerotic morbidity after coronary artery disease and stroke.[2]

Pathophysiology and Risk Factors

PAD is the term used to describe impairment of blood flow to the lower extremities. It is a progressive condition and results from any etiology causing an occlusion or stenosis of the lower limb arteries. Most commonly, the impaired blood flow is a result of atherosclerotic disease. Although much less common, there are nonatherosclerotic causes of PAD (**Box 1**).[3]

Atherosclerosis is a complicated physiologic phenomenon involving several highly interrelated processes, including lipid disturbance, platelet activation and thrombosis, endothelial dysfunction, inflammation, oxidative stress, vascular smooth muscle activation, altered matrix metabolism, and genetic factors.[4] It is a diffuse and progressive process, with a variable clinical presentation and distribution depending on the regional circulation involved.

A specific set of identifiable risk factors plays an important role in the initiation and acceleration of atherosclerotic lesions. Risk factor assessment remains the primary tool used for atherosclerotic disease screening. Race, age, and gender are the identified significant nonmodifiable risk factors. Smoking, diabetes, hypertension, and dyslipidemia make up the majority of the modifiable risk factors. Only smoking and dyslipidemia have been shown, through prospective controlled studies, to be risk factors where modification alters the development or course of PAD.[1] **Fig. 1** summarizes the influence of identified risk factors on PAD. Diabetes and smoking are the risk factors with the greatest risk of concomitant PAD. In patients with diabetes, for every 1% increase in hemoglobin A_{1c}, there is a 26% increased risk of PAD.[5] The severity of PAD found in smokers tends to increase with the number of cigarettes smoked. Cessation of smoking is associated with a decline in the development of intermittent claudication, a sign of symptomatic PAD.[1]

Box 1
Nonatherosclerotic causes of PAD

Peripheral emboli

Aneurysm thrombosis

Arteritis (Takayasu, thromboangitis obliterans, giant cell arteritis, or polyarteritis nodosa)

Fibromuscular dysplasia

Prior trauma or irradiation injury

Aortic coarctation

Primary vascular tumors

Pseudoxanthoma elasticum

Young patients (advential cyst of popliteal artery, popliteal entrapment, or persistent sciatic artery)

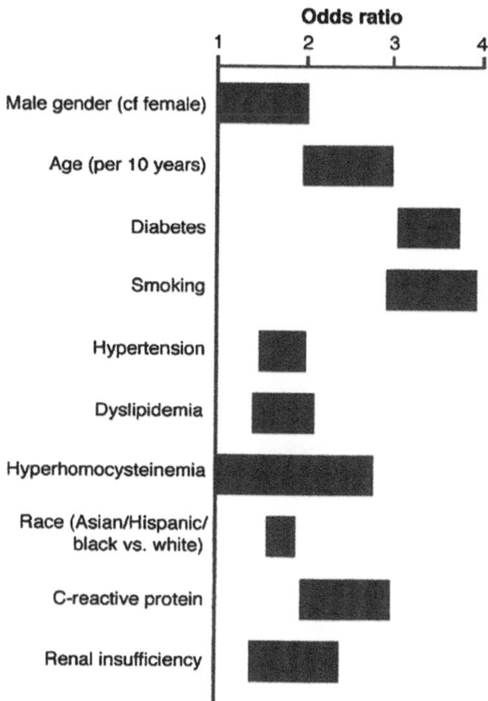

Fig. 1. Approximate range of odds ratios for risk factors for symptomatic PAD. (*From* Norgren L, Hiatt WR, Dormandy JA, et al. Inter-Society Consensus for the Management of Peripheral Arterial Disease [TASC II]. J Vasc Surg 2007;45 Suppl S:S5–67; with permission.)

Current Management

Identification of patients with PAD begins with a data-derived risk factor screening tool, usually in the primary care setting. The primary noninvasive screening test for PAD is the ankle brachial index (ABI). A resting ABI of less than or equal to 0.90 is caused by hemodynamically significant arterial stenosis and is 95% sensitive for detecting arteriogram-positive PAD.[1] Patients with asymptomatic PAD may be medically managed with aggressive risk factor modification, including lifestyle changes, as well as optimal medical management of lipids, hypertension, and diabetes. Smoking cessation is critical and should be medically supported even though long-term success is low. Antiplatelet therapy is indicated for individuals with asymptomatic lower extremity PAD to reduce the risk of adverse cardiovascular events.[6]

Symptomatic PAD ranges in severity from intermittent claudication to critical limb ischemia (CLI). Intermittent claudication is usually diagnosed by a history of muscular leg pain with exercise or ambulation that is relieved by a short rest. CLI defined as ABI less than or equal to 0.40,[7] chronic ischemic rest pain, or clinical evidence of insufficient blood supply (nonhealing ulcers, or gangrene) is the most severe form of PAD and always signals the need for intervention.[8] Patients with CLI experience significant morbidity with cardiovascular event rates surpassing those in patients with symptomatic coronary artery disease.[9] Risk factors and their relative contribution to CLI have been identified (**Fig. 2**).[1] Altering the progression of disease through risk factor modification has not been well studied in patients with CLI. Based on their known cardiovascular morbidity, the same risk factor management optimization in patients with

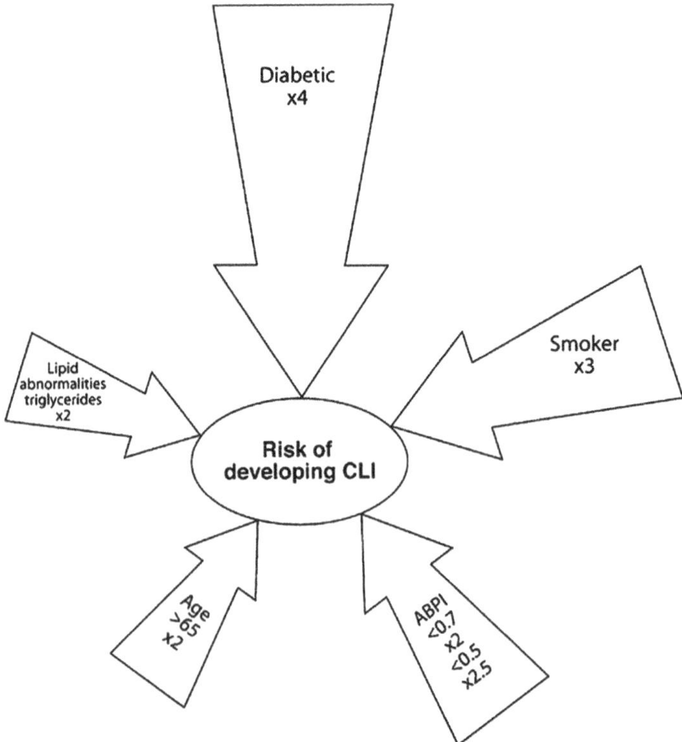

Fig. 2. Magnitude of the effect of risk factors in the development of CLI in patients with PAD. APBI, ankle brachial pressure index. (*From* Norgren L, Hiatt WR, Dormandy JA, et al. Inter-Society Consensus for the Management of Peripheral Arterial Disease [TASC II]. J Vasc Surg 2007;45 Suppl S:S5–67; with permission.)

known coronary artery disease should also be undertaken in this population. A patient with CLI has 15% to 20% mortality and up to a 40% chance of limb loss within 1 year of diagnosis.[10]

It is becoming more difficult to clinically identify the natural history of symptomatic PAD, intermittent claudication, and CLI because most of these patients undergo surgical revascularization. Lower limb revascularization procedures are performed to restore an adequate blood supply to the lower extremities with the goals of improving limb function as well as decreasing pain from claudication. Most commonly these procedures are electively undertaken in conditions of chronic lower extremity vascular insufficiency. The more rare circumstance, intervention for acute lower extremity ischemia, is addressed at the end of this article.

In symptomatic claudication, the need for intervention is based on a patient's disability and functional limitations due to pain from limb ischemia. For many of these patients, treatment is undertaken primarily to prevent lifestyle-limiting claudication and to facilitate an exercise program as ancillary treatment.[11] For patients with CLI, the primary therapeutic goals are relief of pain, wound healing, and preservation of a functional limb, allowing for continued ambulation.[10] A majority of patients require imaging for proper anatomic localization and characterization of the lesion prior to elective operative intervention. Angiography is still considered the gold standard imaging test and most patients undergo full angiography with visualization of the arterial tree from the renal arteries to the pedal arteries as part of their preoperative surgical evaluation.[1]

The appropriate revascularization intervention is a multifactorial decision based on patient comorbidities, anatomic pattern and location of the lesion, flow patterns of inflow and outflow vessels, and availability of autogenous vein graft material. Both endovascular and open surgical techniques are available with anatomic factors exerting a strong influence on surgical decision making.[10] The endovascular techniques for the treatment of patients with lower extremity occlusive disease include balloon angioplasty, stents, stent grafts, and plaque debulking procedures.[1] Surgical options include autogenous or synthetic bypass, endarterectomy, or intraoperative hybrid procedures.[1] Significant progress has been made in endovascular interventions, making the appropriate procedure choice a nuanced decision requiring an in-depth understanding of vascular diseases and the intervention options available. The optimal intervention strategies are debated in the surgical literature and that discussion is beyond the scope of this article. **Fig. 3** provides a simplified framework suggested as a guide for clinical decision making.

PREOPERATIVE EVALUATION

Knowing the risk factors associated with PAD, it is not surprising that significant comorbidities are common in patients presenting for lower extremity revascularization interventions. A majority of these patients are American Society of Anesthesiologists (ASA) III with severe systemic diseases, such as coronary artery disease, hypertension, diabetes mellitus, obstructive lung disease, and cerebrovascular disease, affecting their overall condition for a surgical procedure. A thorough preoperative evaluation is essential to determine their fitness for the proposed surgical procedure as well as to aid in developing an anesthetic plan. The American College of Cardiology and American Heart Association 2007 guidelines for perioperative cardiovascular

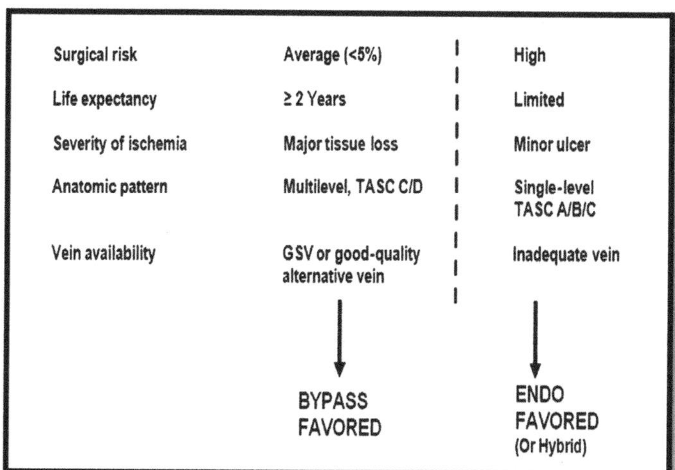

Fig. 3. Key factors involved in selecting the revascularization strategy in CLI. Surgical risk refers to expected 30-day mortality. TASC A/B/C and TASC C/D refer to the anatomical classification of peripheral vascular lesions, with types C/D being more complex lesions. Endo, endovascular therapy; GSV, great saphenous vein. (*From* Conte MS. Critical Appraisal of surgical revascularization for critical limb ischemia. J Vasc Surg 2013;57:8S–13S; with permission.)

evaluation and care for noncardiac surgery rank major vascular surgery as high risk (reported cardiac risk often more than 5%), even in the elective setting.[12]

Functional Capacity

Assessing the functional capacity of these patients may be particularly difficult because their disease process causes lower extremity pain and limits their functional status. Assessment of functional status is particularly important, however, for predicting their postoperative morbidity and mortality. Dosluoglu and colleagues[13] found that ASA III patients with less than 4 metabolic equivalent tasks (METs) functional status had significantly more complications, including myocardial infarction and death, after peripheral revascularization procedures compared with ASA III patients with greater than or equal to 4 METs undergoing similar procedures.

Coexisting Vascular Disease

The risk factors for atherosclerotic PAD are similar to the risk factors that promote atherosclerotic changes in other vascular beds. With this understanding, patients presenting for lower extremity revascularization should have an assessment of the burden of atherosclerotic disease at other locations. As many as 86% of patients have asymptomatic coronary artery disease, 52% have carotid artery disease, and 10% have abdominal aortic aneurysms.[14]

Diabetes Mellitus

Diabetes mellitus is a significant risk factor for the development of PAD, conferring at least a 2-fold increased risk.[15] These patients present with more aggressive PAD with early large vessel involvement and a higher likelihood of amputation. Insulin resistance plays a key role in a list of cardiometabolic risk factors, including hyperglycemia, dyslipidemia, hypertension, and obesity. Additionally, autonomic neuropathies associated with diabetes mellitus can affect the renal vascular bed and lead to hemodynamic instability.

Hypertension

Hypertension is associated with PAD. The relative risk for developing PAD is less for hypertension, however, than for smoking or diabetes. End-organ damage caused by poorly controlled hypertension should be evaluated. Increased cardiovascular lability should be expected in patients with poorly controlled hypertension.

Smoking

Smoking is the most powerful risk factor for the development of PAD and many patients have concomitant chronic obstructive lung disease. Smokers with PAD experience worse disease-specific outcomes, with higher rates of CLI and amputation, higher procedural complications, and increased risk of graft failure.[15]

INTRAOPERATIVE MANAGEMENT

Monitoring

As with most surgical procedures, the choice of monitors is heavily influenced by anesthetic technique, surgical plan, and patient comorbidities. ASA monitoring, as defined by the House of Delegates Committee on Standards and Practice Parameters,[16] should be used during any anesthetic procedure. Noninvasive monitoring, including pulse oximetry and capnography, through the endotracheal tube or sampling line via face mask, is standard.

Accurate ECG monitoring for arrhythmias and myocardial ischemia is particularly important in this population. Many of these patients have coexisting coronary artery disease and are at high risk for intraoperative cardiac events. It has been shown that visual detection of intraoperative ST segment changes is below 50%.[17] Most intraoperative monitors are capable of performing ST segment trend analysis. The use of filters to minimize artifact and the narrow bandwidth of the monitoring mode may, however, adversely affect the sensitivity and specificity of this analysis.[18] Traditionally, after the work of London and colleagues,[19] which showed a sensitivity of 80% for detecting intraoperative ischemic events, leads II and V5 have been monitored intraoperatively. With the addition of another precordial lead, V4, the sensitivity of detecting significant perioperative ischemia is increased to 96%. Lead II is important for the detection of atrial dysrhythmias. More recently, Landesberg and colleagues[20] have re-examined the optimal lead selection and found an 83% sensitivity for significant ischemia while monitoring V4 compared with 76% sensitivity with V5 monitoring. A 95% sensitivity for significant perioperative ischemia was found when 2 precordial leads were monitored. With this information in mind, careful ECG placement and monitoring of 3 leads (II, V4, and V5) is recommended in this population.

Blood pressure monitoring, although required, may be done invasively through direct arterial cannulation or through a noninvasive blood pressure cuff. An argument can be made for continuous blood pressure monitoring in a patient population both sensitive and prone to wide hemodynamic changes. A preinduction arterial line should be considered because induction of anesthesia can be a time with wide hemodynamic variability. During longer procedures or procedures involving heparinization, the access obtained with arterial cannulation may ease necessary laboratory analysis.

For most of lower extremity revascularization procedures, additional invasive monitoring, such as central venous monitors, pulmonary artery catheterization, and transesophageal echocardiography, should not be considered routine. Use of these monitors should be decided on a case-by-case basis considering a patient's comorbidities and the type and duration of the proposed procedure.

Anesthetic Considerations

Patients presenting for peripheral revascularization procedures frequently also have major systemic comorbidities, such as coronary artery disease, hypertension, diabetes, chronic obstructive pulmonary disease, and cerebrovascular disease, making them high-risk surgical candidates. For many years, the literature has debated the anesthetic technique that provides the best outcome for these high-risk patients. Although it has been studied and analyzed, to date there is no single guideline in clinical practice showing that one anesthetic technique provides a significant clinical advantage. Even when the literature is examined through comprehensive meta-analysis, as was done in a recent Cochrane review,[21] the available evidence comparing neuraxial anesthesia and general anesthesia is insufficient to identify significant differences in clinical outcomes.

Cardiac morbidity and mortality

The morbidity and mortality of lower extremity revascularization surgery can be significant. Patients often have severe comorbid conditions, making them complicated surgical candidates. Peripheral vascular surgery is associated with greater cardiac morbidity and overall mortality than other forms of noncardiac surgery.[22] Perioperative myocardial infarction occurs in 4% to 15% of patients undergoing surgery for peripheral vascular disease, and it accounts for greater than 50% of their perioperative mortality.[23] The high incidence of comorbidities and the frequency of complications have led to a discussion about finding an anesthetic solution that minimizes the risk involved in these surgeries. It is accepted that minimizing wide hemodynamic fluctuations during the perioperative period minimizes cardiovascular stress, thereby decreasing perioperative complications. In addition to providing optimal surgical conditions, one of the primary goals of an anesthetic plan for these patients must be to control and minimize the circulatory stresses of surgery in an effort to prevent perioperative cardiovascular and pulmonary complications. It has been hypothesized that using a neuraxial anesthetic technique (ie, spinal or epidural) may allow for improved control of the intraoperative hyperadrenergic state and the postoperative stress response.[24]

After many years of literature debate with studies of weak experimental design that did not produce definitive answers,[25] in 1993, Christopherson and colleagues[26] and the Perioperative Ischemia Randomized Anesthesia Trial Study Group (PIRATS) compared outcomes between general and epidural anesthesia/analgesia techniques in patients undergoing lower extremity revascularization; 100 patients scheduled for elective lower extremity revascularization were randomized to epidural anesthesia/analgesia versus general anesthesia. Cardiac outcomes were comparable in the 2 randomized groups with respect to perioperative death, death within 6 months, nonfatal myocardial infarction within 7 days, and myocardial ischemia. Overall, the trial found that regional and general anesthetic techniques were associated with comparable rates of cardiac morbidity in patients undergoing lower extremity revascularization.

A larger investigation by Bode and colleagues[22] involved 423 participants randomized to general (n = 138), epidural (n = 149), or spinal (n = 136) anesthesia for femoral to distal artery bypass surgery. The study aimed to examine the impact of anesthetic choice on cardiac outcomes in patients undergoing peripheral vascular surgery who had a high likelihood of associated coronary artery disease. The conclusion of the study was that the choice of anesthesia did not significantly influence cardiac morbidity or overall mortality in either an intention-to-treat or type of anesthesia received analysis. After an interim analysis, the investigation was terminated early when it was determined that a large number of participants (24,000) would be required to show a significant difference due to low event rates and similarity in occurrence between the groups.

Most recently, a large observational analysis using the American College of Surgeons National Surgical Quality Improvement Program (NSQIP) database looked at outcomes of lower extremity bypass procedures based on anesthetic type[27]; 5462 inpatient hospital visits involving infrainguinal bypasses for CLI were identified in the analysis. Although a majority of the procedures were performed under general anesthesia (4768), the multivariate analysis demonstrated no significant differences by anesthesia type in the incidence of morbidity (by class or overall) or mortality after infrainguinal bypass. Specifically, the rate of cardiovascular complications was similar between the 2 groups, affecting 2.8% of general anesthesia patients and 2.2% of regional anesthesia patients.

The cumulative effect of the data suggests that the incidence of cardiovascular morbidity and mortality is similar regardless of whether a patient receives a general versus a neuraxial anesthetic technique.[28]

Pulmonary complications

Smoking has been implicated as the single most important risk factor for PAD.[29] Smokers are also more likely to have symptomatic progression of PAD requiring intervention. Therefore, many patients presenting for revascularization procedures can be expected to have pulmonary disease related to their tobacco use. Prevention of perioperative pulmonary complications has been suggested as a benefit of using a neuraxial anesthetic in patients undergoing lower extremity revascularization procedures. No studies comparing neuraxial anesthesia and general anesthesia for lower extremity revascularization have used postoperative pneumonia, respiratory failure, or prolonged intubation as primary endpoints. In a retrospective analysis using the collected Department of Veterans Affairs (VA) NSQIP database, Singh and colleagues[30] found that general endotracheal anesthesia was associated with more cases of postoperative pneumonia (odds ratio 2.2) compared with spinal or epidural anesthesia. Properly administered neuraxial anesthesia allows instrumentation of the airway to be avoided and may be considered in patients with poor preoperative pulmonary function despite a lack of evidence proving its clinical benefit.

Antithrombotic, anticoagulation, and thrombolytic therapy

Antithrombotic or thrombolytic therapy is common in patients presenting for revascularization procedures. Many patients presenting for elective revascularization are on antiplatelet therapy as part of the medical management of their disease or require anticoagulation therapy during the perioperative period. Patients with acute arterial thrombotic disease may be exposed to heparin infusions or thrombolytic therapy. Anesthesiologists must take this into account when considering a neuraxial technique as part of an anesthetic plan as well as when planning for intraoperative blood loss.

Neurologic dysfunction, resulting from hemorrhagic complications, is a reasonable concern when considering a neuraxial technique in patients exposed to antithrombotic or thrombolytic therapy. Although this complication is rare, less than 1 in 150,000 for epidural techniques and 1 in 220,000 for spinal techniques,[31] the consequences can be devastating. Therefore, a careful analysis must be undertaken before using neuraxial techniques in the presence of antithrombotic or thrombolytic therapy. Other risk factors for clinically significant bleeding with neuraxial blockade include increasing age, underlying coagulopathy, difficult needle placement, and an indwelling catheter during sustained anticoagulation.[31]

Antiplatelet therapy Antiplatelet therapy in symptomatic PAD is a key TransAtlantic Inter-Society Consensus (TASC) II recommendation for the medical management of PAD.[1] Some of these patients are maintained only on low-dose aspirin prior to their procedure, but a subgroup of patients are on dual antiplatelet therapy including aspirin and, most commonly, clopidogrel. Antiplatelet medications, including nonsteroidal antiinflammatory drugs (NSAIDs), thienopyridine derivatives (clopidogrel and ticlopidine), and platelet glycoprotein (GP) IIb/IIIa antagonists (abciximab and eptifibatide), exert diverse effects on platelet function. There is no fully accepted test to guide the assessment of the impact of these medications on platelet function. The American Society of Regional Anesthesia and Pain Medicine (ASRA) practice guidelines, relative to the management of patients receiving antiplatelet medications, are as follows:

- NSAIDs seem to represent no added significant risk for the development of spinal hematoma in patients having epidural or spinal anesthesia.
- In patients receiving NSAIDs, recommend against the performance of neuraxial techniques if the concurrent use of other medications affecting clotting mechanisms (oral anticoagulants, unfractionated heparin, or low-molecular-weight heparin) is anticipated early in the postoperative period.
- Suggested time interval between discontinuation of clopidogrel therapy and neuraxial blockade is 7 days.
- If GP IIb/IIIa inhibitors are in use, recovery of platelet function should be documented prior to neuraxial blockade (no specifics on testing requirements).

During the postoperative period, most patients, according to TASC II recommendations, resume or are started on antiplatelet therapy to improve the patency of the revascularization intervention. The postoperative use of antiplatelet therapy should not preclude the use of a single shot neuraxial technique. The risks and benefits of an indwelling catheter should be carefully considered and only left in place if an anesthesiologist is able to ensure frequent neurologic checks once antiplatelet therapy has been started (**Box 2**).

Unfractionated heparin Intraoperative parenteral heparinization (dose range 5000 U to 10,000 U), often used during revascularization procedures, does not preclude the use of neuraxial anesthetic techniques. A recent retrospective review of more than 700 patients undergoing systemic heparinization for cardiopulmonary bypass and receiving neuraxial blockade as part of their anesthetic found no complications related to neuraxial anesthesia.[32] Another large study had similar findings, no epidural hematomas in more than 4000 patients receiving spinal or epidural anesthesia in conjunction with intraoperative heparin during vascular surgery to prevent coagulation during cross clamping of vessels.[33] The ASRA guidelines still caution, however, that neuraxial procedures in the presence of unfractionated heparin may be associated with an increased risk of epidural hematoma, as demonstrated by case series, epidemiologic surveys, and the continued claims in the ASA Closed Claims database.[31] Current ASRA guidelines for neuraxial anesthesia and systemic heparinization include the following:

- Neuraxial blocks should be avoided in patients with other known coagulopathies.
- Time from neuraxial blockade to heparin therapy should exceed 60 minutes.
- Indwelling catheters should be removed 2–4 hours after the last heparin dose with evaluation of patient coagulation status.
- Patients should be monitored closely postoperatively for signs and symptoms of hematoma formation.

Additionally, the guidelines address the postponement of a case for 24 hours if there is a bloody tap or a traumatic regional blockade. There are no clinical data to support this recommendation. The best approach is likely direct communication with the surgeon and a discussion of the risks and benefits of each individual situation.

Thrombolytic therapy Patients are most likely to have received thrombolysis during the management of an acute arterial occlusion. Catheter-directed thrombolysis is often considered a complementary therapy to surgical or percutaneous revascularization, so it is likely that a patient presenting for anesthesia for ALI may have received thrombolytic therapy.[34] The ASRA guidelines recommend against neuraxial anesthesia in patients who have received thrombolytic therapy. There are no specific

Box 2
Recommendation 41: antiplatelet drugs as adjuvant pharmacotherapy after revascularization

Antiplatelet therapy should be started preoperatively and continued as adjuvant pharmacotherapy after an endovascular or surgical procedure (A). Unless subsequently contraindicated, this should be continued indefinitely (A)

Strength of evidence A: based on the criterion of at least one randomized controlled trial as part of the body of literature of overall good quality and consistency addressing the specific recommendation.

From Norgren L, Hiatt WR, Dormandy JA, et al. Inter-society consensus for the management of peripheral arterial disease (TASC II). J Vasc Surg 2007;45:S5A–67A; with permission.

guidelines about how long to avoid neuraxial anesthesia after these drugs have been given or how long to monitor patients who inadvertently receive a neuraxial blockade after thrombolytic therapy.

Graft patency

Early graft failure, occurring within 30 days of the index bypass procedure, is not infrequent and represents a serious complication of lower extremity bypass procedures. Early graft failure is directly associated with an overall poor prognosis.[35] Estimates of the frequency of early graft failure, after open lower extremity bypass procedures, range from 4% to 7%.[36] There are many documented risk factors for early graft failure, including technical factors, thrombosis, conduit adequacy, quality of inflow and outflow vessels, and preoperative functional status.[14] Even the type of anesthesia given during the revascularization procedure has been hypothesized to contribute to the procedure's ultimate success.

There are several hypotheses for why neuraxial anesthesia may improve lower extremity graft patency rates. The sympatholysis provided by neuraxial anesthesia may lead to vasodilation, improved microvascular flow, and possibly reduced arterial vasospasm, theoretically contributing to improved arterial graft patency.[27] Additionally, the prolonged reduction in pain with epidural or spinal anesthesia may decrease the stress response from surgery, attenuating the perioperative inflammatory response and the resultant hypercoagulable state.[37] All of these theoretically contribute to improved graft patency.

Although the theoretic reasoning is logical, the literature findings are not conclusive. Christopherson and colleagues,[26] as part of the PIRATS looking at outcomes between general and regional anesthesia/analgesia, demonstrated a significantly lower rate of graft occlusion among patients receiving an epidural anesthetic technique. This trial found that epidural anesthesia decreased the rate of early graft occlusion from 22% with general anesthesia to 4% with epidural anesthesia. After adjustment for small preoperative differences in heparin administration, age, diabetes, hypertension, smoking history, angina, and previous coronary artery bypass grafting, general anesthesia was found associated with an increased risk of regrafting or thrombectomy. The group also concluded that if the effect on tissue perfusion and graft thrombosis were related to the anesthetic technique, then these events would be temporally related to the administration of the anesthetic and, therefore, would diminish with time. This pattern was observed in this study, with the rate of reoperation in the general anesthesia group much higher in the first few days after surgery, followed by similar reoperation rates in the 2 groups at later times. Based on these results and because no apparent benefit was being conferred by general anesthesia, the clinical monitoring committee terminated the trial early.

Singh and colleagues,[30] analyzing 14,788 patients in the prospectively collected VA NSQIP database, found similar results regarding improved graft patency with neuraxial anesthesia. There was a total of 723 (4.9%) graft failures in the cohort, which is in line with the expected frequency of graft failure for lower extremity arterial bypass. After controlling for confounders using a multivariate model, the odds of graft failure were 43% higher in patients receiving general anesthesia than those receiving spinal anesthesia.

Other studies have not shown the same benefit of neuraxial anesthesia relative to graft patency. Pierce and colleagues,[38] in a retrospective analysis of a randomized prospective trial designed to study cardiac outcomes after vascular surgery, found that the type of anesthetic given for femoral to distal artery bypass does not significantly affect 30-day graft occlusion. More recently, Ghanami and colleagues,[27] in a retrospective analysis of 5463 procedures, using the NSQIP database, found no difference in the rates of graft failure between neuraxial and general anesthetic techniques. A similar conclusion was reached by Wiis and colleagues.[39] In a retrospective study of the Danish Vascular Registry, examining 938 lower extremity revascularization procedures on 822 patients, they found that the type of anesthesia did not influence the 7-day graft failure rate. With the hypothesis that "the protective epidural effect" would be even greater on smaller vessels, a subanalysis was performed on femorodistal procedures. There was no difference between the 2 anesthesia types in the subgroup either. Also important to this study is that all participants underwent an in situ bypass procedure using autogenous vein graft material. This implies that the ability of the graft to vasodilate and constrict remains intact and the vessel is sensitive to sympathetic stimulation; therefore, the suspected benefits of epidural anesthesia (sympathetic blockade) should have been evident.

Early graft failure is a devastating complication of lower extremity bypass and clearly multifactorial in origin. Given the available evidence, however, it is not obvious that the type of anesthetic influences this outcome. Factors, such as patient preference, coexisting disease, local expertise, and practice patterns, should continue to govern anesthetic choice for these procedures.

POSTOPERATIVE CONCERNS

The postoperative location for many of these patients depends on their intraoperative course as well as the need for hemodynamic and peripheral vascular monitoring. Postoperative care should be multidisciplinary, with a focus on continued hemodynamic stability, excellent pain control, and frequent verification of adequate limb perfusion. The risk of cardiac morbidity in these high-risk patients continues into the postoperative period. Simultaneous with the highest incidence of adverse cardiac events, catecholamine levels increase gradually in the first 48 hours after surgery.[40] Stable hemodynamics and pain control may decrease the catecholamine surge and improve postoperative myocardial complications.

Although there were not conclusive data to show benefits of neuraxial anesthesia over general anesthesia during the intraoperative phase, there may be some benefit to epidural analgesia during the postoperative period. Recently a large meta-analysis, including 125 trials and 9044 patients, examined the impact of epidural analgesia on mortality and morbidity after a range of surgical procedures.[41] All patients had a general anesthetic for intraoperative management. The meta-analysis found that concomitant epidural analgesia reduces postoperative mortality and improves a multitude of cardiovascular, respiratory, and gastrointestinal endpoints compared with patients receiving systemic analgesia (**Fig. 4**).

With careful consideration, in light of anticoagulation and antithrombotic therapies commonly used in revascularization procedures, postoperative epidural analgesia may be beneficial in reducing some of the postoperative morbidity associated with these procedures.

ACUTE LIMB ISCHEMIA

Acute limb ischemia (ALI), referring to an abrupt cessation of flow to an extremity, is a vascular emergency requiring urgent revascularization in an effort to avoid limb amputation. ALI is associated with high morbidity, including bleeding requiring transfusion, limb amputation, fasciotomy, and renal insufficiency.[1] Thirty-day mortality rates are greater than 25% after embolectomy for ALI.[42]

Patients present with symptoms similar to lower extremity compartment syndrome: pain, pallor, pulselessness, paresthesia, and paralysis. The potential causes of ALI are

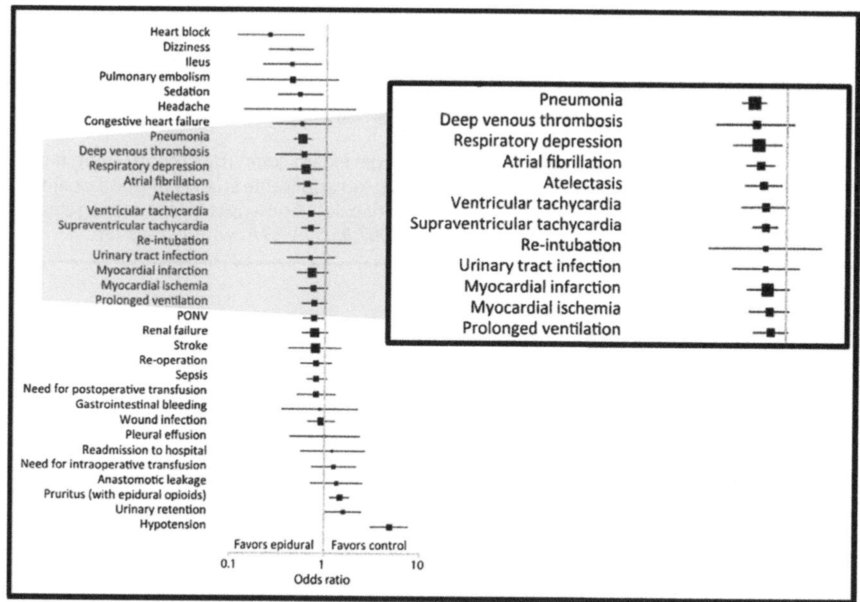

Fig. 4. Impact of epidural analgesia on postoperative mortality and morbidity. Control indicates systemic opioid-based analgesia. PONV, post operative nausea and vomiting. (*From* Popping DM, Elia N, Van Aken HK. Impact of epidural analgesia on mortality and morbidity after surgery. Ann Surg 2014;259(6):1056–67; with permission.)

most commonly arterial thrombus, in situ arterial thrombosis in the setting of advanced chronic arterial occlusive disease, and major arterial trauma. The timing of presentation is related to the cause and severity of ischemia. Patients with traumatic injuries or acute arterial thrombosis present within hours of ischemic onset, whereas those with native thrombosis or reconstruction occlusions tend to present at later time periods due the presence of collateral arterial flow. For most presentations, restoration of flow is established through 2 primary treatment options: (1) catheter-based thrombolytic therapy with adjunctive mechanical thrombectomy or (2) surgical thrombectomy with as-needed adjunctive bypass or endarterectomy.[43]

From an anesthetic standpoint, the major challenge with these procedures is their emergent nature. Often there is little time to adequately evaluate patients and optimize their medical comorbidities without further compromising the ischemic extremity. A brief targeted history should address the basics, including allergies, current medications, airway assessment, cardiac and pulmonary history, and other significant comorbidities. A reasonable set of preoperative laboratory studies and an ECG in appropriate populations is also warranted.

According to the TASC II guidelines for the management of PAD parenteral anticoagulation is indicated for all patients presenting with ALI (**Box 3**).[1]

Therapeutic parenteral anticoagulation (ie, heparin infusion) during the preoperative period makes general anesthesia (as opposed to neuraxial anesthesia) the most reasonable choice in these patients.

Monitoring beyond standard ASA monitors should be chosen based on patient comorbidities and other operative circumstances. Most of these patients, other than those with acute traumatic injuries, likely have systemic vascular disease and should, therefore, be considered high risk for perioperative cardiac complications. Finally,

Box 3
Recommendation 31: anticoagulation therapy in ALI

Immediate parenteral anticoagulant therapy is indicated in all patients with ALI. In patients expected to undergo imminent imaging/therapy on arrival, heparin should be given (C)

Strength of evidence C: based on evidence obtained from expert committee reports or opinions and/or clinical experiences of respected authorities (ie, no applicable studies of good quality).

From Norgren L, Hiatt WR, Dormandy JA, et al. Inter-Society Consensus for the Management of Peripheral Arterial Disease (TASC II). J Vasc Surg 2007;45:S5A–67A; with permission.

reperfusion of the ischemic limb may lead to profound acid-base disturbances, which are often difficult to treat and require aggressive resuscitation.

SUMMARY

Patients presenting for revascularization procedures of the lower extremity are often complex patients with significant systemic comorbidities leading to multiple perioperative complications. Unfortunately, the data to date do not show the benefit of one anesthetic technique over another for these procedures. Neuraxial techniques may be desirable in some patients, especially those with significant pulmonary disease; however, there is no clear evidence that neuraxial anesthesia minimizes cardiac morbidity or improves graft patency for these procedures. There is some affirmation that postoperative epidural analgesia may reduce cardiac morbidity; however, the use of an indwelling epidural catheter must be carefully considered in a population also treated with systemic anticoagulation or antithrombotic therapy. Anesthesiologists should appreciate the procedural goals and the impact and risks of patient systemic comorbidities and use this understanding to establish an anesthetic plan that maximizes hemodynamic stability and optimal pain control throughout the perioperative period.

REFERENCES

1. Norgren L, Hiatt WR, Dormandy JA, et al. Inter-society consensus for the management of peripheral arterial disease (TASC II). J Vasc Surg 2007;45 Suppl S: S5–67.
2. Gerald F, Fowkes R, Rudan D, et al. Comparison of global estimates of prevalence and risk factors for peripheral artery disease in 2000 and 2010: a systematic review and analysis. Lancet 2013;382:1329–40.
3. Abdulhannan P, Russell DA, Homer-Vanniasinkam S. Peripheral arterial disease: a literature review. Br Med Bull 2012;104:21–39.
4. Faxon D, Fuster V, Libby P, et al. Atherosclerotic Vascular Disease Conference Writing Group III: pathophysiology. Circulation 2004;109:2617–25.
5. Selvin E, Marinopoulos S, Birkenblit G, et al. Meta-analysis: glycosylated hemoglobin and cardiovascular disease in diabetes mellitus. Ann Intern Med 2004; 141:421–31.
6. Anderson JL, Haperin JL, Albert NM. Management of patients with peripheral artery disease (compilation of 2005 and 2001 ACCF/AHA guideline recommendations). Circulation 2013;127:1425–43.
7. Belch JJ, Topol EJ, Agnelli G, et al. Critical issues in peripheral arterial disease detection and management: a call to action. Arch Intern Med 2003;163:884–92.
8. Varu VN, Hogg ME, Kibbe MR. Critical limb ischemia. J Vasc Surg 2010;51: 230–41.

9. Caro J, Miggliaccio-Walle K, Ishak KJ, et al. The morbidity and mortality following a diagnosis of peripheral arterial disease: long-term follow-up of a large database. BMC Cardiovasc Disord 2005;5:14.
10. Conte MS. Critical appraisal of surgical revascularization for critical limb ischemia. J Vasc Surg 2013;57:8S–13S.
11. Bettmann MA, Dake MD, Hopkins LN, et al. Atherosclerotic Vascular Disease Conference: Writing Group VI: revascularization. Circulation 2004;109:2643–50.
12. Fleisher LA, Beckman JA, Brown KA, et al. ACC/AHA 2007 guidelines for perioperative cardiovascular evaluation and care for noncardiac surgery: executive summary: a report of the American College of Cardiology/American Heart Association task force on practice guidelines. Circulation 2007;116:1971–96.
13. Dosluoglu H, Wang J, DeFranks-Anain L, et al. A simple subclassification of American Society of Anesthesiology III patients undergoing peripheral revascularization based on functional capacity. J Vasc Surg 2008;47:766–73.
14. Ghansah JN, Murphy JT. Complications of major aortic and lower extremity vascular surgery. Semin Cardiothorac Vasc Anesth 2004;8:335–61.
15. Tattersall MC, Johnson HM, Mason PJ. Contemporary and optimal medical management of peripheral arterial disease. Surg Clin North Am 2013;93:761–78.
16. Standards for Basic Anesthetic Monitoring. ASA House of Delegates Committee on Standards and Practice Parameters. Surg Clin North Am 2013;(90):761–78.
17. Mangano DT, Hollenberg M, Fegert G, et al. Perioperative myocardial ischemia in patients undergoing noncardiac surgery–I: incidence and severity during the 4 day perioperative period. The Study of perioperative Ischemia (SPI) Research Group. J Am Coll Cardiol 1991;17:843–50.
18. Fleisher LA. Real-time intraoperative monitoring of myocardial ischemia in noncardiac surgery. Anesthesiology 2000;92:1183–8.
19. London MJ, Hollenberg M, Wong MG, et al. Intraoperative myocardial ischemia: localizations by continuous 12 lead electrocardiography. Anesthesiology 1988; 69:232–41.
20. Landesberg G, Mosseri M, Wolf Y, et al. Perioperative myocardial ischemia and infarction: identification by continuous 12-lead electrocardiogram with online ST-segment monitoring. Anesthesiology 2002;96:264–70.
21. Barbosa FT, Juca MJ, Castro AA, et al. Neuraxial anesthesia for lower-limb revascularization. Cochrane Database Syst Rev 2013;(7):CD007083.
22. Bode RH, Lewis KP, Zarich SW, et al. Cardiac outcome after peripheral vascular surgery. Comparison of general and regional anesthesia. Anesthesiology 1996; 84:3–15.
23. Mangano DT. Perioperative cardiac morbidity. Anesthesiology 1990;72:153–81.
24. Tuman KJ, Ivankovich AD. Regional anesthesia is better than general anesthesia for lower extremity revascularization. J Cardiothorac Vasc Anesth 1994; 8:114–7.
25. Gelman S. General versus regional anesthesia for peripheral vascular surgery, is the problem solved? Anesthesiology 1993;79:415–8.
26. Christopherson R, Beattie C, Frank S, et al. Perioperative morbidity in patients randomized to epidural or general anesthesia for lower extremity vascular surgery. Anesthesiology 1993;79:422–34.
27. Ghanami RJ, Hurie J, Andrews JS, et al. Anesthesia-based evaluation of outcomes of lower-extremity vascular bypass procedures. Ann Vasc Surg 2013; 27:199–207.
28. Wesner L, Marone LK, Dennehy KC. Anesthesia for lower extremity bypass. Int Anesthesiol Clin 2005;43:93–109.

29. Selvarajah S, Black JH, Malas MB. Preoperative smoking is associated with early graft failure after infrainguinal bypass surgery. J Vasc Surg 2014;59(5):1308–14.
30. Singh N, Sidawy AN, Dezee K, et al. The effects of the type of anesthesia on outcomes of lower extremity infrainguinal bypass. J Vasc Surg 2006;44:964–70.
31. Horlocker TT, Wedel DJ, Rowlingson JC, et al. Regional anesthesia in the patient receiving antithrombotic and thrombolytic therapy. Reg Anesth Pain Med 2010; 35:64–101.
32. Weiner MM, Rosenblatt MA, Mittnacht AJ. Neuraxial anesthesia and timing of heparin administration in patients undergoing surgery for congenital heart disease using cardiopulmonary bypass. J Cardiothorac Vasc Anesth 2012;26: 581–4.
33. Liu SS, Mulroy MF. Neuraxial anesthesia and analgesia in the presence of standard heparin. Reg Anesth Pain Med 1998;23:157–63.
34. van den Berg JC. Thrombolysis for acute arterial occlusion. J Vasc Surg 2010;52: 512–5.
35. Singh N, Sidawy AN, Dezee KJ, et al. Factors associated with early failure of infrainguinal lower extremity arterial bypass. J Vasc Surg 2008;47:556–61.
36. Soma G, Greenblatt DY, Nelson MT, et al. Early graft failure after infrainguinal arterial bypass. Surgery 2014;155:300–10.
37. Rosenfeld BA, Beattie C, Christopherson R, et al. The effects of different anesthetic regimens on fibrinolysis and the development of postoperative arterial thrombosis. Anesthesiology 1993;70:435–43.
38. Pierce ET, Pomposelli FB, Stanley GD, et al. Anesthesia type does not influence early graft patency or limb salvage rates of lower extremity arterial bypass. J Vasc Surg 1997;25:226–33.
39. Wiis JT, Jensen-Gadegaard P, Altintas U, et al. One-Week postoperative patency of lower extremity in situ bypass graft comparing epidural and general anesthesia: retrospective study of 822 patients. Ann Vasc Surg 2014;28:295–300.
40. Raby KE, Brull SJ, Timimi F, et al. The effect of heart rate control on myocardial ischemia among high-risk patients after vascular surAnesth Analggery. Anesth Analg 1999;88:477–82.
41. Popping DM, Elia N, Van Aken HK. Impact of epidural analgesia on mortality and morbidity after surgery: systematic review and meta-analysis of randomized controlled trials. Ann Surg 2014;259(6):1056–67.
42. Ellard L, Djaiani G. Anaesthesia for vascular emergencies. Anaesthesia 2013; 68(Suppl 1):72–83.
43. Blecha MJ. Critical limb ischemia. Surg Clin North Am 2013;93:789–812.

Intraoperative Management of Carotid Endarterectomy

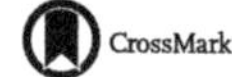

Andrey Apinis, MD*, Sankalp Sehgal, MD, Jonathan Leff, MD

KEYWORDS

- Carotid endarterectomy • Carotid stenosis • Intraoperative management
- Neurophysiologic monitoring

KEY POINTS

- Carotid endarterectomy (CEA) is an effective and low-risk intervention for prevention of stroke in symptomatic and asymptomatic patients with severe carotid stenosis.
- CEA can be safely performed under either general anesthesia (GA) or locoregional anesthesia (LRA) (cervical plexus block) with similar mortality and morbidity.
- Neurologic monitoring (electroencephalography [EEG], stump pressure [SP] measurement, evoked potentials [EPs], transcranial Doppler [TCD], or cerebral oximetry) is advantageous when utilizing general anesthesia.
- Significant complications consist of strokes (mostly embolic), myocardial ischemia, and postoperative hypertension.
- In rare cases, hypertension progresses to cerebral hyperperfusion syndrome (CHS).

INTRODUCTION

First reports on the surgical treatment of cerebrovascular atherosclerosis date to the early 1950s.[1] Initial outcomes were not promising due to suboptimal surgical technique, which consisted of an end-to-end carotid anastomosis. With time, surgical technique has evolved and subsequent outcomes have improved.[2] Enthusiasm for CEA was revived after results of the first randomized trials were published in the 1990s. With more recent data, CEA has emerged as an effective measure for the prevention of stroke in patients with symptomatic and asymptomatic severe carotid artery stenosis.[3] In terms of the 5-year risk of ipsilateral ischemic stroke, randomized

Conflict of Interests: Dr J. Leff has consulted for Casmed Systems. The authors declare that there are no additional financial, consultant, institutional, or other relationships that might have led to bias or a conflict of interests regarding the publication of this article.
Cardiothoracic Anesthesiology, Montefiore Medical Center, Albert Einstein College of Medicine, 111 E 2 10th Street, Bronx, NY 10467, USA
* Corresponding author.
E-mail address: Aapinis@montefiore.org

Anesthesiology Clin 32 (2014) 677–698
http://dx.doi.org/10.1016/j.anclin.2014.05.008 **anesthesiology.theclinics.com**
1932-2275/14/$ – see front matter

controlled trials examining CEA versus medical treatment have shown significant benefit to surgical intervention. The advantage of surgery is most significant in patients with greater than 70% internal carotid artery (ICA) stenosis and recent symptoms.[4]

Two large randomized trials, the North American Symptomatic Endarterectomy Trial and the European Carotid Surgery Trial, highlighted the benefit of surgical intervention. The combined results of these trials, as outlined in a meta-analysis, showed an absolute risk reduction for the combined outcome of death and subsequent stroke. Given the benefits that surgery offers beyond medical management, the number of CEA procedures continues to increase. This article explores the anesthetic management and considerations of patients undergoing CEA.

GENERAL VERSUS LOCOREGIONAL ANESTHESIA

Adequate surgical anesthesia for CEA can be achieved by both GA and LRA. A combination of deep and superficial cervical plexus blocks was historically used for this purpose; however, there are data to support that superficial block alone with supplemental wound infiltration and sedation[5] is equally effective. It is beyond the scope of this article to describe the technical aspects of performing regional anesthesia for CEA. This information is highlighted in an article by Guay[5] that describes the relevant aspects of performing regional anesthesia for CEA.

The most significant benefit of performing CEA under LRA is constant neurologic assessment of patients. This becomes crucial during the period of carotid cross-clamping, where cerebral circulation is potentially compromised. The onset of new neurologic symptoms should immediately alert the anesthesiologist and surgeon to possible ipsilateral brain hypoperfusion. These cerebral symptoms should prompt an adjustment in surgical technique, involving ipsilateral shunt insertion. Other real or perceived benefits of LRA include a reduction of postoperative respiratory complications secondary to the avoidance of endotracheal intubation. Additional benefits include a lower incidence of postoperative hypertension that may decrease the incidence of CHS[6,7] and the avoidance of the physiologic stress of induction and intubation, which may help minimize cardiac complications.

There are, however, many disadvantages when choosing LRA over GA. Most intraoperative strokes are the result of thromboembolism, not hypoperfusion, and occur during reperfusion.[8] The intraoperative placement of a shunt, which may occur during GA or LRA, does not diminish the incidence of thromboembolic stroke. In addition, should major neurologic deterioration or excessive sedation occur during LRA, establishing airway patency in an agitated or disinhibited patient under the surgical drapes can be difficult. Also, sudden movement of an awake patient during surgery is undesirable and dangerous. Moreover, as with any regional anesthetic, cervical plexus block may provide inadequate anesthesia or analgesia, necessitating an unplanned conversion to GA, or cause systemic toxicity (1.4% and 4.4%, respectively).[9]

Regardless, more patients with advanced systemic disease are referred for CEA and the avoidance of GA seems an attractive option. This view was encouraged by the results of studies claiming a reduced incidence of cardiovascular and respiratory complications in patients having general surgery procedures under neuraxial anesthesia.[10] Guay,[5] based on retrospective data, asserted that patients who had CEA performed under LRA had a decreased incidence of strokes, myocardial infarction (MI), death, respiratory impairment, and wound infection.

The General Anaesthesia Versus Local Anaesthesia for Carotid Surgery (GALA) study was a large, multicenter randomized controlled trial seeking to provide a definitive answer on which type of anesthesia is preferable for CEA. Its intended size was

5000 patients but only 3526 were enrolled from 1999 to 2007. Results were mostly inconclusive and demonstrated a nonsignificant trend toward a lower rate of neurologic complications and higher rate of myocardial ischemia in the LRA arm. There was no difference in quality of life at 1 month postoperatively between the 2 groups.[9] The investigators concluded that there is insufficient evidence to advise for or against either type of anesthesic plan for routine CEA.

The GALA study results were collaborated by an article by Sideso and colleagues,[11] published in 2011. In this retrospective, nonrandomized single-center study, results from 383 patients (260 of them performed under LRA) were analyzed. They found a higher incidence of stroke in the GA group and a higher incidence of myocardial ischemia and death in the LRA group; however, neither of these differences reached statistical significance. As with the GALA study, a higher but nonstatistically significant incidence of cranial nerve damage was noted in the LA group.[11] Vaniyapong and colleagues,[12] in a recent Cochrane review on the benefits of local versus GA for CEA, reported similar results. The investigators did not find a statistically significant difference in the rate of stroke, MI, or death between GA and LRA.

In summary, the authors agree with the conclusion of the GALA trial and of Vaniyapong and colleagues[12] that there is insufficient evidence to support LA over GA. The choice of anesthetic should be based on patient preference, experience of the perioperative team, institutional resources, and individual factors (patient's ability to cooperate, neck anatomy, and so forth). Surgeons and anesthesiologists should be proficient in both techniques, realizing the advantages and limitations of each, and use the technique best suited for a particular patient.

INDUCTION AND MAINTENANCE OF GENERAL ANESTHESIA

All patients presenting for CEA should have standard American Society of Anesthesiologists monitors—ECG, pulse oximetry, end-tidal CO_2, and temperature. Considering the high prevalence of coronary artery disease (CAD) in this population and significant risk of myocardial ischemia and MI, a 5-lead ECG is strongly advised. Most anesthesiologists prefer invasive blood pressure monitoring over noninvasive, which allows for a prompt response to unanticipated blood pressure swings. During carotid clamping, if induced hypertension is used, arterial blood pressure monitoring allows for precise titration of vasopressors. The presence of an arterial catheter can be even more important in the immediate postoperative period when hypertension can quickly progress to CHS. In this situation, exact knowledge of arterial blood pressure and its response to vasodilators help achieve the predefined range of blood pressure.[13] The placement of 2 peripheral intravenous catheters allows for one to be used for vasoactive infusions and the other for maintenance fluid and boluses. Anticipated blood loss is usually minimal and central venous or large-bore peripheral access is rarely necessary.

The use of a sedative-hypnotic medication is often necessary when providing anesthesia in patients undergoing CEA with a regional technique. Even with a successful regional block, some degree of sedation is useful to alleviate patient anxiety and discomfort. There are several medications that can be used to safely achieve patient comfort (midazolam, fentanyl, morphine, propofol, and dexmedetomidine); however, excessive sedation should be avoided. Overly aggressive use of opioid and sedative-hypnotic medications can result in respiratory depression and possible hemodynamic instability. Also, heavy sedation resulting in altered mental status and lack of patient cooperation complicates the assessment of a patient's neurologic status—the very goal of conducting the CEA under LRA.

If GA is chosen for CEA, endotracheal intubation as opposed to LMA is generally preferable. Medications chosen for induction of anesthesia should be based on a patient's overall condition, preoperative risk profile, physician preference, and institutional routine. Ketamine should be used with caution because of its ability to increase cerebral metabolism, stimulate release of adrenergic substances, and interact with neurologic monitoring. The use of large doses of opioids may result in delayed emergence from anesthesia and impair postprocedural neurologic assessment.

Maintenance of GA is typically achieved by administering inhalational volatile agents, supplemented with opioids and neuromuscular blockers. Neurologic monitoring includes EEG, somatosensory evoked potentials (SSEPs), and motor evoked potentials (MEPs). All of these may be used during CEA to assess the adequacy of cerebral perfusion. Intravenous medications and inhaled anesthetics can alter the interpretation of the data derived from the EEG, SSEPs, or MEPs. Total intravenous anesthesia is preferred when EP monitoring is used, because it has minimal impact on the assessment of neurologic signals during the monitoring phase. In the authors' experience, a combination of propofol and remifentanil is a reliable choice to maintain a sufficiently deep and steady level of anesthesia with a predictable fast onset and offset while having minimal impact on EP monitoring. If MEPs are used, avoiding the continued use of neuromuscular blockers is preferred.

Wide swings in blood pressure in the perioperative period are common and are related to the atherosclerotic plaque commonly located in the area of the carotid sinus. The baroreceptors on the carotid sinus are involved in the regulation of blood pressure and heart rate. During years of plaque formation on the intimal layer of the carotid bifurcation, these receptors have decreased contact with blood flow and gradually alter their sensitivity to stimuli. Manipulations on the carotid sinus during dissection may, therefore, elicit hemodynamic instability, often accompanied by rhythm changes.[14] Sudden bradycardia is frequently seen, although rarely affecting outcome.[15] Extremely low heart rates can significantly decrease cardiac output and compromise organ perfusion, and it is prudent to have positive chronotropic agents (atropine or glycopyrrolate) available if significant bradycardia results in hemodynamic instability. In the past, infiltration of the carotid sinus with local anesthetic was believed to attenuate the bradycardia associated with operative site manipulation. This is controversial, however, and local infiltration may even contribute to a higher incidence of postoperative hypertension.[16] Examination of randomized control trials assessing local infiltration has failed to show a benefit with regard to hemodynamic stability during CEA.[17]

One of the most crucial events during CEA is cross-clamping of the carotid artery. It is preceded by systemic heparinization, with a goal activated clotting time of 200 to 250 seconds. Carotid cross-clamping allows a surgeon to remove the atherosclerotic plaque while working in a nonpulsatile and bloodless field. After the procedure, the anesthesiologist and surgeon must weigh the risk and benefit of heparin reversal with protamine.

It is desirable to verify neurologic intactness prior to extubation; however, coughing and bucking should be avoided, which may precipitate surgical bleeding. After extubation, patients are usually transferred to a postanesthesia care unit for close observation of neurologic status and cardiovascular function, unless ICU admission is advisable due to a patient's perioperative risk profile or specific postoperative concerns.

CAROTID CROSS-CLAMPING AND SHUNTING

As a consequence of carotid cross-clamping, antegrade carotid blood flow to the ipsilateral cerebral hemisphere is acutely interrupted; afterward, all oxygen delivery is dependent on collateral flow from the circle of Willis (**Fig. 1**). If collateral flow is inadequate, cerebral hypoperfusion ensues, increasing the possibility of stroke. Several strategies exist to attenuate malperfusion during carotid cross-clamping. Administration of supplemental oxygen and the use of phenylephrine or norepinephrine to artificially elevate the mean arterial blood pressure (and, hence, cerebral perfusion pressure) are nonspecific interventions that theoretically increase blood flow and oxygen delivery to the cerebral tissues.[18]

The efficacy of these simple maneuvers is questionable. Giustiniano and colleagues[19] analyzed the relationship between arterial blood pressure and cerebral oximetry as a surrogate of cerebral oxygenation during CEA. They concluded that there is no correlation between the trends of these 2 variables and advocate abandoning induced hypertension. Some institutions have a neuroprotective protocol that consists of induced hypertension, systemic hypothermia, and administration of large doses of a hypnotic medication (propofol or barbiturate). This protocol can be activated if signs of inadequate cerebral blood flow are detected by the onset of neurologic symptoms in an awake patient or changes observed during neuromonitoring.[20]

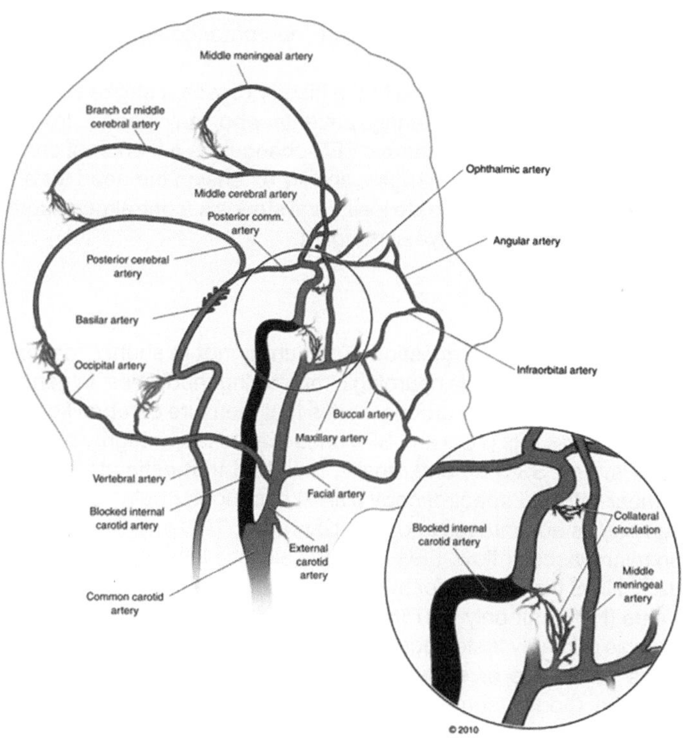

Fig. 1. Demonstrates collateral blood flow with carotid stenosis and the normal arterial cerebral anatomy. (*From* Erickson KM, Cole DJ. Carotid artery disease: stenting vs endarterectomy. Br J Anaesth 2010;105(Suppl 1):i36; with permission.)

The most popular strategy for addressing hypoperfusion during carotid clamping is to insert a shunt to bypass the arteriotomy site and enable partial antegrade blood flow from the common carotid artery (CCA) to the ICA. Although the concept seems logical, additional manipulation is not without potential consequences and may increase the incidence of embolic stroke.[21] The presence of a shunt does not diminish the embolic load and increases the risk of embolism from air, debris, or elements of the plaque.[20] Other complications related to shunting include damage of the arterial wall,[22] acute carotid occlusion,[23] and intimal tears.[24] Insertion of the shunt adds complexity to the case and may be technically difficult. As a result, the incidence of local complications—cranial nerve damage, infection, and wound hematoma—is increased[24,25] with shunt placement. Moreover, shunting does not guarantee restoration of blood flow,[24] while at the same time increasing the likelihood of late complications—CHS[26] and restenosis.[24]

Nevertheless, certain patients are susceptible to cross-clamp induced ischemia. Studies performed during CEA under LRA consistently demonstrate that 10% to 15 % of patients develop acute neurologic symptoms shortly after carotid clamping and benefit from shunt placement.[3,27–29] Individual surgeons and institutions have different approaches to this problem. Some never use shunting whereas others place shunts routinely.[25] AbuRahma and colleagues[23] in their review on shunting observed an overall stroke rate of 1.4% with routine shunting and 2% with routine nonshunting. Currently, most neurosurgeons place a shunt selectively, basing their decision on new neurologic symptoms in an awake patient. In patients undergoing GA, the decision is contingent on a low SP or changes in neuromonitoring indicating cerebral malperfusion.

A Cochrane review from 2009 found that a history of recent stroke and contralateral carotid stenosis are markers to identify patients who may benefit from shunting.[4] Ballotta and colleagues,[30] using ischemic EEG changes as a marker of cerebral hypoperfusion, concluded that these changes, and by extension the need for a shunt, can be predicted by prior stroke, moderate ipsilateral stenosis, contralateral carotid occlusion, and patients with preoperative symptoms.

NEUROLOGIC MONITORING

A more definitive answer to the question "To shunt or not to shunt?" can be obtained using some of the many available neurologic monitoring modalities. In general, all neuromonitoring can be divided in 3 groups—ones that measure cerebral flow or pressure in the large cerebral vessels (TCD and SP); ones that assess integrity of cerebral function (EEG, MEPs, and SSEPs); and, finally, monitors that estimate cerebral oxygen metabolism (near-infrared spectroscopy [NIRS] and jugular bulb saturation).[31]

Each group has its advantages and disadvantages. TCD and SP do not provide information on microvascular flow. EEG is technically challenging and has a 41% false-negative rate.[27] NIRS technology for evaluating cerebral ischemia has a good negative predictive value (NPV) but only a 47% positive predictive value (PPV).[32] Accuracy of each method was primarily tested against the gold standard of LRA and it is not known if cutoff values for awake or slightly sedated patients are transferable to patients under GA,[33] even though some data suggest they can be used interchangeably (**Table 1**).[34]

Electroencephalography

EEG represents electrical activity of the brain. A detailed description of this diagnostic modality is beyond the scope of this article, but in the perioperative period no EEG

Table 1
Overview of the various types of monitors used during carotid endarterectomy to detect cerebral ischemia, thromboembolism, or both

Neurologic Monitor	Description	Advantages	Disadvantages
Awake testing	Using simple tasks for a patient to perform to assess the signs for cerebral ischemia	Direct monitor of neurologic function	As discussed previously for performing CEA under RA
TCD	A Doppler probe is placed on the petrous temporal bone, allowing measurement of MCA flow.	Monitors both flow and emboli, used inter- and postoperative period	• Operator dependent • Placement is near the surgical site. • Acoustic window is not found in 10%–20% of patients.
SP	The SP distal to the carotid clamp reflects the perfusion pressure around the circle of Willis.	Specific measure of cerebral ischemia	• Nonsensitive measure of cerebral ischemia • Cannot identify emboli
EEG	EEG is affected by cerebral ischemia. Raw and processed (spectral array) data can be used.		• Measurement only reflects cortical and not deeper structure. • Difficult to interpret • GA can alter the signal. • Cannot identify emboli
SSEPs	EEG is recorded after a stimulus, thus reflects the cortex and deeper structure activity.	May be useful if baseline EEG is abnormal	• GA can alter the signal. • Thought no more sensitive or specific compared with EEG • Cannot identify emboli
NIRS	NIRS measures arterial venous and capillary oxygenation, producing an rSo_2 value.	High NPV for cerebral ischemia	• Poor PPV • Frontal lobe sensors • Interference from noncerebral blood flow and light • Cannot identify emboli

Adapted from Ladak N, Thompson J. General or local anesthesia for carotid endarterectomy? Contin Educ Anaesth Crit Care Pain 2012;12(2):93.

changes are observed with cerebral blood flow decreasing from normal—approximately 50 mL/100 g/min—to 22 mL/100 g/min.[35] With further reduction to 18 mL/100 g/min, observing signs of brain ischemia can be expected.[36] Ischemic EEG changes occurring after carotid cross-clamping could indicate potential cerebral ischemia and warrant shunt insertion (**Fig. 2**).

When comparing EEG changes against the gold standard—new neurologic symptoms under regional anesthesia—Hans and Jareunpoon[27] found a disturbingly high incidence of false-negative results (40.6%). The incidence of false-positive results in their series was 1.0%. The investigators concluded that EEG as a monitor of cerebral ischemia in the setting of CEA has poor sensitivity—59.4%. One of the possible explanations for the observed low sensitivity is that EEG reflects only processes in the cerebral cortex and does not detect the electrical activity of deeper brain structures.

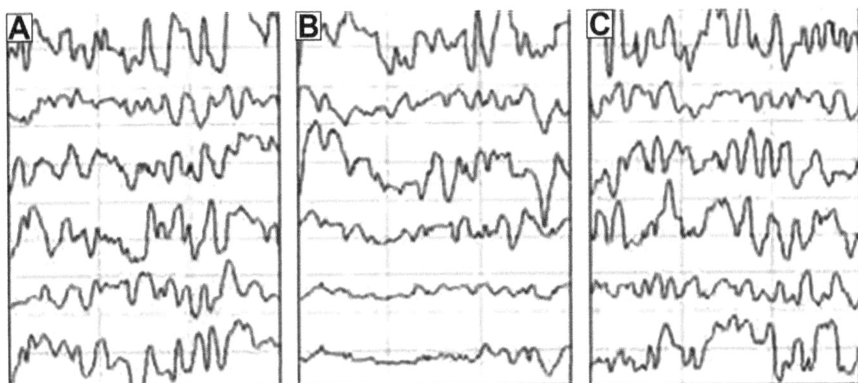

Fig. 2. Raw EEG during carotid endarterectomy (*A*) before an ischemic event, (*B*) during an ischemic event, and (*C*) during recovery from an ischemic event. (*From* Liu H, Giorgio A, Williams E, et al. Protocol for electrophysiological monitoring of carotid endarterectomies. J Biomed Res 2010;24(6):463.)

EEG reveals nonspecific regional physiologic imbalances that can be a consequence of many factors—interrupted blood flow, hypoxia, and systemic hypotension. In addition, the EEG signal is affected by certain anesthetics and hypothermia.[35] Utilization of this modality necessitates trained personnel for the interpretation of raw data and avoidance of certain anesthetic medications and it adds complexity to the logistics of the operating room.

Arguably, the most important limitation of EEG is the need for a continual interpretation of raw data. Commercially available monitors of anesthesia depth use sophisticated processing software that significantly simplifies the reading of EEG information. Although not specifically marketed for the purposes of neurologic monitoring during CEA, ease of application, compact size, familiarity to anesthesia providers, and uncomplicated reporting scale make these monitors an attractive alternative to multichannel EEG. Working with a bispectral index monitor (BIS) (Covidien, Dublin, Ireland), Estruch-Perez and colleagues[37] found that a decrease of BIS value by 14% has an 82% sensitivity and 90% specificity for diagnosing cerebral ischemia. These devices have a 30- to 60-second delay in reporting, and they are capable of detecting changes only if they occur in frontal lobes.[38]

Evoked Potentials—Somatosensory Evoked Potentials and Motor Evoked Potentials

Measuring EPs is another diagnostic modality used to monitor functional neurologic status. SSEPs are the most common type of EP monitored in the setting of CEA and utilize stimuli of known intensity, duration, and frequency applied to the median (more common) or tibial nerve. After stimulation, the amplitude and latency of the signal is measured over the cerebral cortex. Therefore, EPs reflect the integrity of the deep cerebral structures. A decrease in the signal for the median nerve points to hypoperfusion in the watershed of middle cerebral artery (MCA). Tibial nerve signal abnormalities are indicative of hypoperfusion of the areas supplied by the anterior cerebral artery.[39,40] Most investigators accept a 50% decrease in the EP signal amplitude as indicative of ischemia.[25,27,33,41]

Moritz and colleagues[33] compared the accuracy of multiple neurologic monitoring methods to assess potential cerebral ischemia in 48 patients during CEA under LRA.[33] For SSEP monitoring, they reported a sensitivity of 81% and specificity of

57%. Two of 8 patients who needed shunt placement based on the clinical symptoms did not have any changes in SSEP amplitude recorded after the carotid artery was cross-clamped. On the other hand, changes in TCD and NIRS were diagnostic for ischemia in these 2 patients. False-negative results with SSEP monitoring have been reported by other investigators as well.[42–44]

The underlying mechanism for this decreased accuracy may be focal ischemia in the internal capsule.[45] Monitoring MEPs as opposed to SSEPs should theoretically overcome this issue. Many investigators believe that MEPs are more sensitive to cerebral ischemia than SSEPs.[46] To monitor MEPs, the cerebral cortex is stimulated via transcranial electrodes and a motor response in the contralateral extremity (upper and lower) is recorded. Uchino and colleagues[46] demonstrated the feasibility of this technique in 20 patients undergoing CEA. They found a consistent correlation between a 50% amplitude decrease in MEPs and a 20% drop in NIRS during cerebral ischemia. In the retrospective multicenter study of 600 CEA patients, Malcharek and colleagues[45] reported no false-negative MEPs results whereas SSEPs had a 1.5% rate of false-negative results. In this study, 75% or more decrease in MEP amplitude was considered significant for ischemia.

As discussed previously, after both common and external carotid arteries are clamped antegrade flow distal to the clamp decreases. In this situation, perfusion pressure in the vessels supplying the ipsilateral hemisphere is supported via collaterals from the circle of Willis. Measuring pressure just distal to the clamp site (SP, termed *carotid back pressure* in old articles) was advocated for many years as a way to ensure adequate blood flow. It is performed by inserting a small needle in the distal CCA and transducing the pressure. Advantages of this monitoring method are that it provides a direct gauge of cerebral perfusion, does not require sophisticated equipment with specially trained personnel, and is cost effective and compact. There is no level 1 evidence, however, that adequate perfusion pressure (as defined by SP) ensures brain functional integrity, and the critical value of SP is not known.

Some investigators measure systolic arterial pressure whereas others rely on mean arterial pressure.[27] It is unclear which number to use as a reference point for measuring SP.[33] Most importantly, different arbitrary ischemic thresholds, with a range from 25 mm Hg[47] to 50 mm Hg,[48,49] are reported in the literature, with a range of 40 mm Hg to 45 mm Hg being the target for not placing a shunt. Moritz and colleagues,[33] in their study on 48 patients under LRA, found that a cutoff value of 40 mm Hg for SP produced a sensitivity of 100% and specificity of 75% for the development of neurologic complications. Hans and Jareunpoon,[27] in similar circumstances, reported a specificity of 97.4% and sensitivity of 56.8%. In their study, specificity and sensitivity changed to 98.6% and 29.8%, respectively, if 50 mm Hg was chosen as a cutoff value for SP. As with other monitoring modalities, it is not known if results obtained under local anesthesia are transferable to patients having GA for CEA.[24]

Aburahma and colleagues[50] found that an SP of 40 mm Hg is an adequate threshold for shunting under GA. Harada and colleagues[51] evaluated the validity of an SP threshold of 50 mm Hg against EEG changes in 140 CEA cases performed under GA. According to their study, this cut off value has a sensitivity of 89%, a 96% NPV and a 36% PPV.

Considering the significant variations in designs, methods, and settings of the different studies, it is difficult to come to a definitive conclusion on the current role of SP measurement during CEA. Most likely, as with other monitoring modalities, it will continue to be used by surgeons who are comfortable interpreting SP values.

Transcranial Doppler

TCD serves as an alternative to SP in estimating cerebral blood flow. A 2-MHz probe is applied to the ipsilateral temporal area and a depth of 45 to 55 mm is insonated. The Doppler shift of the returning signal reflects flow in the MCA. TCD does not measure blood flow directly.[35] Instead, it provides information about the maximal blood velocity. In ultrasound physics, flow is the product of velocity in the vessel and cross-sectional area of the vessel. In most cases, however, large cerebral arteries, such as the MCA, have a fixed diameter[52] and maximal velocity corresponds well with the flow.

TCD is unique among other neurologic monitors due to its usefulness beyond detecting cerebral hypoperfusion during carotid clamping.[52] Its importance is underscored by purely ischemic events responsible for only a minority of neurologic damage after CEA, whereas a majority of strokes are caused by thromboembolic phenomena.[24] TCD can contribute to the safe conduct of CEA in multiple ways: (1) it provides quantitative auditory information about the embolic load during carotid dissection; (2) it can be used to ensure that the flow level remains above a predefined ischemic threshold after clamping; (3) if a shunt is used, TCD may be used to confirm that flow through the shunt is adequate; and (4) it can identify patients with acute postoperative thrombosis.[53]

TCD also has the advantage of being compact and easily interpreted. It is operator dependent[26] but less so than EEG or EPs. Its main disadvantage is the difficulty in obtaining a reliable Doppler signal in a high proportion of patients. This failure rate is reported from 10% to 15%[54–56] to 21%.[33] In addition, the ischemic threshold for TCD is not known. Moritz and colleagues,[33] in their study of 48 CEA patients under LRA, found that reduction of MCA velocity (MCAV) to 50% of baseline provides 100% sensitivity and 86% specificity; using a 70% reduction in velocity changes the specificity to 100% at the expense of decreasing the sensitivity to 78%. Also, in the setting of LRA, Ali and colleagues[3] found that a decrease in mean velocity of 50% or more has sensitivity and specificity of 75% for need of shunting. They calculated PPV and NPV as 37.5% and 93.9%, respectively. With such a remarkable range of reported values, the exact place of TCD in preventing ischemic complications after carotid clamping currently is unknown (**Fig. 3**).

Near-Infrared Spectroscopy

One of the newest modalities available for monitoring neurologic status during CEA is NIRS. Measuring oxygenation in the frontal cerebral cortex provides an estimate of oxygen balance and theoretically should detect reduction of flow below a critical level. Via 2 adhesive pads on the forehead, NIRS uses multiple wavelengths of light (660–940 nm) to calculate regional cerebral oxygen saturation (rSo_2). The amount of light absorbed by oxyhemoglobin and deoxyhemoglobin at specific wavelengths is inversely related to the amount of light received at a photodetector. In the presence of increased amounts of oxyhemoglobin, more light is absorbed and less is reflected to the photodetector, a concept known as the Beer-Lambert law.

The current commercially available devices have 2 light detectors for each light emitter and allow the subtraction of extracranial tissue for a more accurate rSo_2 value. Despite the technological advances, concern for contamination of the signal by extracerebral interference exists.[24,33] The distance from the light source to the detector determines spatial resolution. By having 1 light detector proximal, the more superficial vasculature can be accounted for and theoretically not contaminate the cerebral oximeter value (**Fig. 4**).

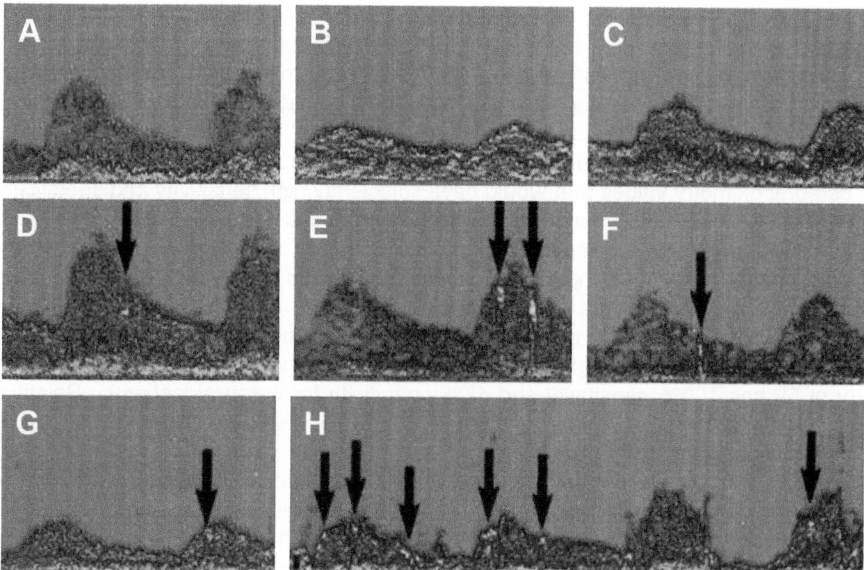

Fig. 3. TCD diagnosis of on-table carotid thrombosis, which was diagnosed during wound closure. (*A*) Beginning of operation (MCAV = 48 cm/s). (*B*) The ICA is clamped (MCAV = 24 cm/s). (*C*) Shunt opened (MCAV = 42 cm/s). (*D*) Flow restored after endarterectomy (MCAV = 68 cm/s). (*E*) First emboli detected in ipsilateral MCA (*arrows*). (*F*) After further embolization, MCAV declines to 43 cm/s. (*G*) MCAV has fallen to 27 cm/s, which is similar to when the ICA was clamped, indicating that the ICA is either occluded or nearly occluded. (*H*) The wound has been reopened and gentle handling of the ICA triggers the release of numerous emboli into the ipsilateral MCA, causing MCAV to increase to 40 cm/s. After reopening the ICA, the endarterectomy zone was almost completely occluded with fresh thrombus. After removal of the thrombus, there was no evidence of any underlying technical error. (*From* Gaunt ME. Diagnosis of early postoperative carotid artery thrombosis determined by transcranial Doppler scanning. J Vasc Surg 1994;20(1):105; with permission.)

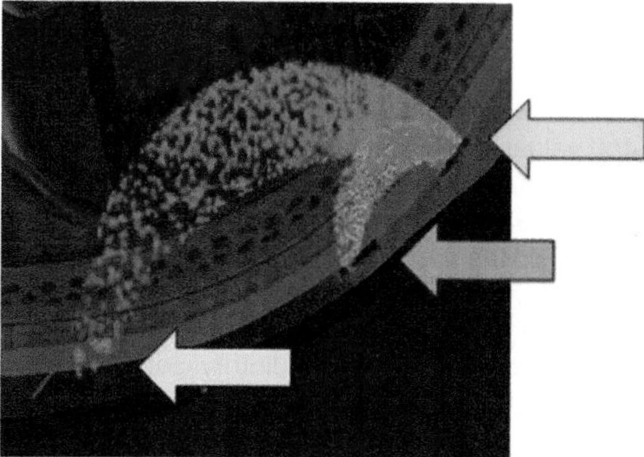

Fig. 4. The *yellow arrow* is the point of light emission (laser or LED). The near-field detector is marked by an *orange arrow* and the far field detector is marked by a *white arrow*. (*Courtesy of* CAS Medical Systems, Brandford, CT; with permission.)

The appeal of NIRS stems from many factors. It is portable, simple to interpret without special training, inexpensive, and easily applicable. NIRS represents, however, a region of cerebral tissue oxygen saturation at the frontal gray matter and ischemia in other parts of the brain can potentially be missed. Another limitation is that cerebral oximetry may be inaccurate over an area of previous infarction.[46] With these shortcomings in mind, many attempts were undertaken to establish an absolute or relative decrease in cerebral oximetry values that would have sufficiently high sensitivity and specificity in determining cerebral ischemia so that surgical technique could be optimized.

Few studies were performed under regional anesthesia using clinical examination as a gold standard for verifying the accuracy of cerebral oximetry. Moritz and colleagues[33] analyzed different neurologic monitors in 48 awake patients. For NIRS, they used the INVOS 3100 cerebral oximeter (Somanetics, Troy, Michigan). It was determined by these investigators that an absolute threshold value for cerebral oximetry of 59 has 100% sensitivity and 47% specificity for cerebral ischemia. Relative changes had better specificity—a decrease of 20% from baseline value was 83% specific (with 83% sensitivity as well).

Ritter and colleagues,[29] using the INVOS 4100 device on 100 CEA patients, found that a drop in rSo_2 more than 19% after carotid clamping has sensitivity of 100% and specificity of 98% (yielding PPV of 82% and NPV of 100%) for the need of shunt insertion. On the other hand, using the same INVOS device in a similar setting and with a 19% drop from baseline as the ischemic threshold, Stilo and colleagues[57] reported only 60% sensitivity and 25% specificity. Another study by Ali and colleagues[3] compared accuracy of TCD and cerebral oximetry to the awake testing in detecting cerebral ischemia on 49 CEA patients. Their results showed 75% sensitivity and 97.5% specificity for a 20% decrease in rSo_2 (corresponding to PPV of 85.7% and NPV of 95.2%).

As with other neuromonitoring modalities, there is a question if the results obtained on awake patients are applicable to patients under GA.[33] Several studies from as early as 2000 compared NIRS technology with the older and more established monitoring techniques. For example, Manwaring and colleagues,[58] while validating decreases in cerebral oximetry values (rSo_2) (INVOS system) against SP below 40 mm Hg, reported 76.3% sensitivity and 81.1% specificity for a 15% baseline reduction and 57.9% sensitivity with 86.8% specificity for a 20% reduction in rSo_2.

For the same critical SP, Tambakis and colleagues[59] found good correlation with a 21% decrease in cerebral oximetry at 1 minute and 10% at 5 minutes after carotid clamping. Mauermann and colleagues[60] used the Equanox 7600 monitor (Nonin Medical, Plymouth, Minnesota) and compared changes occurring during CEA with ischemic changes on EEG. They used a 5% absolute and a 10% relative reduction, respectively, of the cerebral oximetry value as predetermined cutoff points. They reported that both cutoff values had 75% sensitivity to predict cerebral ischemia. Specificity was 74% for an absolute change and 84% for the negative change in rSo_2. Both parameters had high NPV (98%) but low PPV (14% and 21%, respectively).[60] A larger study by Pennekamp and colleagues[61] compared the accuracy of both TCD and NIRS with EEG in the CEA setting. They found that a 16% decrease in rSo_2 had PPV of 76% and NPV of 99% and is the optimal threshold for NIRS.

At first glance, these results seem contradictory and confusing. Several factors could have contributed to the lack of uniformity. These studies were performed on different devices each with its own proprietary hardware and software. As opposed to EEG or EP, there is no normal cerebral oximetry value and interindividual variations are considerable.[24] A more reasonable approach would be to look at the relative changes in cerebral oximetry that follow carotid cross-clamping (see **Fig. 2**). Most recent studies discuss 19% and 21% reductions as possible ischemic thresholds; however, older studies have used lower thresholds, ranging from 11.7%[62] to 13%.[63] As a consequence of these conflicting results, different investigators have opposing views on the usefulness of NIRS as a tool to detect and prevent cerebral ischemic complications during CEA. Although some investigators note high sensitivity and specificity of cerebral oximetry[29] and find it more accurate than TCD,[3] others state that NIRS technology cannot be used reliably[55] and its role in this setting is modest.[57] There are anecdotal reports on NIRS able to detect acute carotid thrombosis during surgery and verify shunt patency after its placement.[64] Unique among other modalities, NIRS sensors can be easily left in place after actual procedure is completed and monitoring be continued in the postoperative period. Promising data exist on cerebral oximetry predicting development of CHS (**Fig. 5**).

Neuromonitoring Conclusion

There are no definitive recommendations on whether routine, selective, or no shunting should be used during CEA. A Cochrane review of shunting during CEA from 2009 states that routine shunting offers no significant benefit on stroke rate compared with no shunting. The article also points out that no randomized data are available to compare selective shunting with no shunting. The investigators conclude that current evidence is insufficient to either support or disprove the use of routine or selective shunting in CEA.[22]

Similar uncertainty exists regarding the methods of neurologic monitoring. Many years have been spent in search of an ideal neuromonitor, with hundreds of articles devoted to this question. Yet the definite answer is still missing. AbuRahma and colleagues[23] performed a meta-analysis of all CEA trials published from 1990 to 2010.

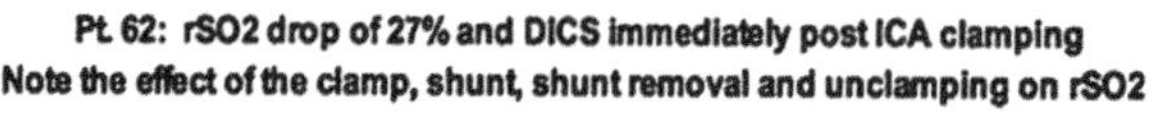

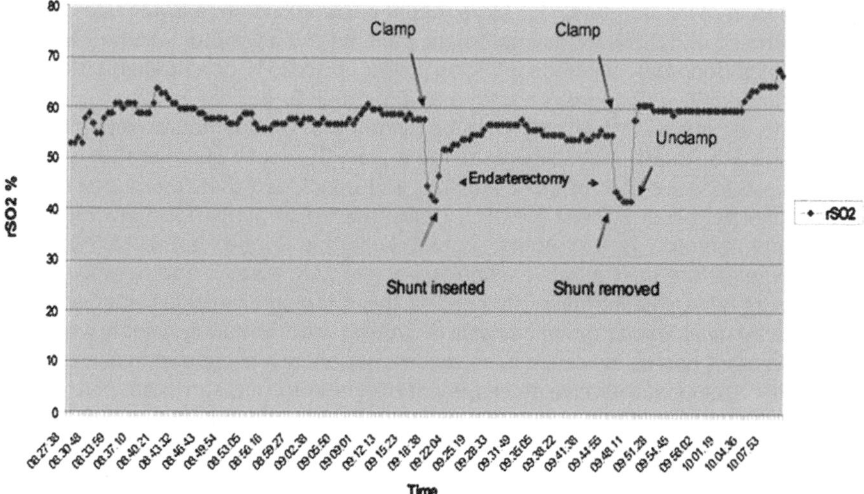

Fig. 5. The effects of shunting and cross-clamping on rSo_2 in a patient undergoing CEA. DICS, deterioration in conscious status. (*From* Rittera JC, Greenb D, Slim H, et al. The role of cerebral oximetry in combination with awake testing in patients undergoing carotid endarterectomy under local anesthesia. Eur J Vasc Endovasc Surg 2011;41(5):601; with permission.)

They found the incidence of perioperative stroke 1.6% if shunt placement is selected based on EEG, 4.8% if based on TCD, 1.6% for SP, and 1.8% for SSEPs. Guay and Kopp[65] in their meta-analysis of studies comparing different types of cerebral monitoring systems with clinical brain monitoring, concluded that individually none of the monitors can detect cerebral ischemia as accurately as performing CEA under LRA.

This conclusion seems collaborated by Rerkasem and Rothwell, who write in their Cochrane review that "no one method of monitoring in selective shunting has been shown to produce better outcomes."[4] Accuracy may be enhanced by combining different monitors. The review by Guay and Kopp[65] states that the best combination for neuromonitoring would be SP with TCD or EEG. Although the search for a perfect monitoring technique is ongoing, different anesthesiologists, neurosurgeons, vascular surgeons, and institutions have adopted varying strategies to minimize hypoperfusion-related cerebral complications with similar results. In the meantime, application of these monitoring modalities during CEA have developed beyond diagnosing hypoperfusion after carotid clamping, with TCD used to approximate embolic load and both TCD and NIRS used to predict development of CHS (see **Table 1**).

COMPLICATIONS

Complications related to CEA can be broadly divided into 3 categories: periprocedural systemic complications, periprocedural local complications, and late complications.[66] Periprocedural systemic complications include hemodynamic lability, stroke, MI, death, and CHS. Periprocedural local complications include carotid thrombosis, wound hematoma and infection, and cranial nerve damage. Late complications include re-stenosis and false aneurysm.[66] Immediate systemic complications present the most impressing challenges to anesthesiologist and are discussed in detail later.

Stroke

Stroke is one of the most dreaded complications of CEA, with an incidence of 3% to 5% reported in older literature.[20,67] More recent publications state lower rates: 1.1% for symptomatic and 0.5% for asymptomatic patients.[68] If asymptomatic new MRI lesions are included, this incidence is higher[69] and up to 25% of all patients develop subtle neurocognitive changes 1 month after the procedure.[70,71]

A majority of intraoperative strokes are caused by thromboembolic events during reperfusion.[8] Rockman and colleagues[72] analyzed 38 acute perioperative strokes that occurred in the series of 2024 patients and concluded that thromboembolism was responsible for 24 strokes (65.2%), clamp-related ischemia for 5 (13.2%), and intracerebral hemorrhage for another 5 (13.2%). Of the 24 strokes, 4 (10.5%) were deemed unrelated to the operative technique or site. Because embolism or hypoperfusion occurs during the intraoperative period, the neurologic deficit usually becomes apparent after awakening from anesthesia (if GA was used) or during surgery when using LRA. In other cases, the onset of symptoms secondary to hypoperfusion may be delayed.[22,73] Late postoperative development of symptoms after an intact period may be related to uncommon sources of strokes like ICA thrombosis, dissection or occlusion.[64]

Carotid Thrombosis

Carotid thrombosis at the site of intervention is rare (less than 1% according to[67]) and leads to cerebral ischemia. It is known that a high embolic load precedes the development of thrombosis.[35] Based on this observation, Naylor and colleagues[53] included in their institutional protocol routine extended use of TCD monitoring and administration of dextran-40 to high-risk patients. This strategy helped to virtually eliminate postoperative thrombotic complications. Later, both routine TCD monitoring and dextran therapy were abandoned in favor of routine dual antiplatelet therapy with similar successful results.

Local Hematoma and Infection

As with any surgical intervention, there is always a risk for development of infection or hematoma at the site of the wound. Although length of incision for CEA is only a few centimeters, the proximity of the trachea imparts significant risk should a hematoma occur. It is reported that wound hematoma develops in 5% to 8 % of cases[2] and 1% to 3% of all CEA require re-exploration for bleeding.[13] Meticulous hemostasis during surgery should minimize the risk for hematoma formation. Intensive monitoring in the immediate postoperative period will enable rapid intervention at the first signs of an expanding hematoma. If symptoms of airway compromise are observed, urgent endotracheal intubation is warranted. In the gravest situation, opening some of the skin sutures allows blood collected in the wound to drain and helps relieve pressure on the airway.

Cranial Nerve Injury

Owing to the anatomic proximity of the carotid sheath, the following cranial nerves can be injured during the procedure: mandibular branch of the facial nerve, recurrent laryngeal nerve (branch of the vagus nerve), and hypoglossus and glossopharyngeal nerves. These injuries are usually minor and transient.[66] The surgical literature also discusses parotid fistulas and injury to the sympathetic plexus as potential albeit rare local complications.[2]

Myocardial Ischemia and Infarction

Patients with significant atherosclerosis of cerebral vessels are expected to have a similar atherosclerotic burden in other vascular beds, and a high incidence of myocardial ischemia and MI after CEA has been observed. According to an article by Hertzer and colleagues[74] published in 1986, up to 35% of patients referred for CEA were found to have severe CAD. Researchers from the north american symptomatic carotid endarterectomy trial collaborators (NASCET) group (1991) reported a 0.9% rate for MI[75]; however, many patients with severe systemic disease were not eligible for an enrollment in this trial. In the carotid revascularization endarterectomy versus stenting trial (CREST) trial, the incidence of MI was 2.3% in the CEA arm, which included a more real-world population.[76] A Cochrane review from 2013 analyzed outcomes of 11 CEA studies conducted from 1989 to 2010 and found the incidence of perioperative MI 0.5%.[12] It is possible that if more sensitive biochemical assays for markers of myocardial damage were used on the asymptomatic patients, the resulting rate of myocardial ischemia would be higher.[77] Most MIs after CEA are non-ST segment elevation MIs and are classified as type II, meaning that the acute imbalance of myocardial oxygen supply/demand is caused by a mechanism different from acute coronary occlusion. This type of MI also confers a poor long-term prognosis.[77]

MI after CEA, with a reported incidence of 1.1%,[12,67] is a major cause of death. It is not unusual for patients to have some degree of hemodynamic instability after CEA, and although both hypotension and hypertension can occur, most cases involve hypertension. If hypotension is detected, the underlying cause should be sought aggressively (myocardial ischemia, medication error, or significant postoperative bleeding). In a majority of cases, the hypertensive response is transient and lasts only for few hours.[78] Although preexisting hypertension seems to be a logical cause, some patients who develop hypertension postoperatively have normal blood pressure prior to surgery. Some data suggest that performing CEA under local as opposed to GA minimizes the incidence of postoperative hypertension, albeit at the expense of a higher incidence of intraoperative hypertension.[6,7] It is likely that impaired baroreceptor reactivity immediately after removal of an atheroma from the carotid artery has the greatest contribution to the hemodynamic instability after CEA.[78]

Elevated blood pressure after CEA predisposes patients to a variety of serious complications. Increased aortic wall tension leads to an increased afterload and thus higher myocardial work and oxygen consumption. These conditions predispose patients to myocardial ischemia and arrhythmias. In addition, the risk of wound hematoma is increased with elevated blood pressure.

Postoperative hypertension is strongly associated with the development of CHS (discussed later). Due to the potential complications of postoperative hypertension, the management of this condition should be prompt and effective. Up to 40% of CEA patients require antihypertensive therapy after the procedure.[15] Some institutions use strict protocols aimed at the aggressive treatment of hypertension after CEA and are contigent on a patient's symptoms, ability to tolerate oral medications, and personal history. Typical protocols include the use of labetalol, hydralazine, and nitroglycerin to control hypertension and mitigate adverse events.[53] Naylor and colleagues[53] assert that implementation of a protocol significantly reduced the incidence of CHS, intracranial hemorrhage and major cardiac events; however, their data also revealed a higher incidence of contralateral ischemic stroke in the same time period.

Cerebral Hyperperfusion Syndrome

The presence of severe extracranial cerebral atherosclerosis alters baroreceptor reactivity and autoregulation in the cerebral vasculature. CEA succeeds in removing the atherosclerotic plaque; however, the physiologic response does not immediately normalize. CHS has an incidence of 3% to 5% after CEA[79,80] and may occur in other cerebral revascularization procedures.[79] CHS typically occurs in the first few hours after the procedure, although late-onset presentation up to 4 weeks has been reported.[79] The symptoms include ipsilateral headache, facial and eye pain that in severe cases can progress to seizures, intracerebral hemorrhage, brain edema, and coma.[52,64] Mortality from CHS is reported to be 40%.[81] Besides altered baroreceptor reactivity and vasomotor paralysis, other factors that potentially contribute to the development of CHS include intraoperative ischemia,[82] severe preoperative ipsilateral,[25] and contralateral[81] stenosis.

Considering the rare occurrence and high mortality of CHS, it is important to identify potential CHS patients early.[54] Many post-CEA patients experience some degree of cerebral hyperperfusion not classified as CHS. A small subset of patients who experience at least a 2-fold increase in cerebral blood flow on the affected side compared with their baseline value are at particularly high risk.[79] It has been determined that 40% of these patients develop neurologic symptoms and progress to CHS.[26] TCD, with an ability to accurately measure blood velocity (and thus estimate the cerebral flow), seems a promising monitoring tool for detecting this condition. Controversies exist as to what constitutes a normal postoperative velocity. Liu and colleagues[83] postulate that increase in cerebral blood velocity found after the conclusion of surgery is more predictive for the development of CHS than the more traditionally used similar increase seen immediately after the release of carotid cross-clamp. These results seem collaborated with a study by Pennekamp and colleagues.[26]

TCD, although considered a gold standard for the diagnosis of CHS, is not an ideal monitoring device. As discussed previously, this modality is unable to obtain a reliable signal in a significant proportion of patients. Cerebral oximetry can serve as an attractive alternative to TCD in diagnosing CHS. Earlier works by Ogasawara and colleagues[84] identified postoperative increase in rSo_2 of 5% or more as a risk factor for CHS, with a 10% increase 100% sensitive and specific. In a series of 151 CEA patients, Pennekamp and colleagues[54] found that patients who developed CHS had an increase in NIRS values of 3% immediately after clamp release and 7% postoperatively. They concluded that NIRS is a reliable method to exclude patients at risk. A combination of NIRS and TCD may have a better PPV. Early identification of patients at risk, as well as aggressive antihypertensive treatment with close monitoring of neurologic status, minimizes the development of this lethal condition.[66]

CONCLUSIONS AND FUTURE DEVELOPMENTS

The future direction of carotid surgery may involve a less invasive approach. The use of angioplasty and carotid stents has been explored in several studies. With the emergence of endovascular stents, percutaneous treatment of severe carotid stenosis has become available. This procedure is almost always performed under conscious sedation and offers the potential for less postoperative hemodynamic disturbance and lack of local, surgical complications. Several trials explored the feasibility and risk profile of the endovascular approach. In terms of acute neurologic morbidity, initial results were not promising; however, cardiovascular morbidity might have been reduced. It is possible that with further advancement in stent design and deployment technology (ie, embolic protectors) as well as better patient selection and provider experience, carotid artery stenting will surpass CEA in efficacy and safety.

Currently, carotid artery stenting is recommended as an alternative treatment to CEA for symptomatic patients with severe carotid stenosis and an expected low rate of periprocedural complications.[68] Certain patient-specific anatomic considerations (location of the stenosis, previous neck surgery, and radiation) help determine which approach is better suited for particular patients.[85] In the future, advances in pharmacologic research related to cerebrovascular disease may allow medical treatment alone to become the standard of care for asymptomatic patients with carotid stenosis.[86]

REFERENCES

1. Eastcott HH, Pickering GW, Rob CG. Reconstruction of internal carotid artery in a patient with intermittent attacks of hemiplegia. Lancet 1954;267:994–6.
2. Curtis JA, Johansen K. Techniques in carotid surgery. Neurosurg Focus 2008; 24:E18.
3. Ali AM, Green D, Zayed H, et al. Cerebral monitoring in patients undergoing carotid endarterectomy using a triple assessment technique. Interact Cardiovasc Thorac Surg 2011;12(3):454–7.
4. Rerkasem K, Bond R, Rothwell PM. Local versus general anaesthesia for carotid endarterectomy. Cochrane Database Syst Rev 2004;(2):CD000126.
5. Guay J. Regional anesthesia for carotid surgery. Curr Opin Anaesthesiol 2008; 21(5):638–44, 2.
6. Eibes TA, Gross WS. The influence of anesthetic technique on perioperative blood pressure control after carotid endarterectomy. Am Surg 2000;66(7):641–7.
7. Scuderi PE, Prough DS, Davis CH Jr, et al. The effects of regional and general anesthesia on blood pressure control after carotid endarterectomy. J Neurosurg Anesthesiol 1989;1(1):41–5.
8. Krul JM, van Gijn J, Ackerstaff RG, et al. Site and pathogenesis of infarcts associated with carotid endarterectomy. Stroke 1989;20:324–8.

9. GALA Trial Collaborative Group, Lewis SC, Warlow CP, Bodenham AR, et al. General anaesthesia versus local anaesthesia for carotid surgery (GALA): a multicentre, randomised controlled trial. Lancet 2008;372(9656):2132–42. http://dx.doi.org/10.1016/S0140-6736(08)61699-2.
10. Rodgers A, Walker N, Schug S, et al. Reduction of postoperative mortality and morbidity with epidural or spinal anaesthesia: results from overview of randomised trials. BMJ 2000;321:1493.
11. Sideso E, Walton J, Handa A. General or local anesthesia for carotid endarterectomy–the "real-world" experience. Angiology 2011;62(8):609–13.
12. Vaniyapong T, Chongruksut W, Rerkasem K. Local versus general anaesthesia for carotid endarterectomy. Cochrane Database Syst Rev 2013;(12):CD000126. http://dx.doi.org/10.1002/14651858.CD000126.pub4.
13. Kresowik TF, Bratzler D, Karp HR, et al. Multistate utilization, processes and outcomes of carotid endarterectomy. J Vasc Surg 2001;33(2):227–35.
14. Hirschl M, Kundi M, Blazek G. Five-year follow-up of patients after thromboendarterectomy of the internal carotid artery: relevance of baroreceptor sensitivity. Stroke 1996;27:1167–72.
15. Wong JH, Findlay JM, Suarez-Almazor ME. Hemodynamic instability after carotid endarterectomy: risk factors and associations with operative complications. Neurosurgery 1997;41:35–41 [discussion: 41–3].
16. Al-Rawi PG, Sigaudo-Roussel D, Gaunt ME. Effect of lignocaine injection in carotid sinus on baroreceptor sensitivity during carotid endarterectomy. J Vasc Surg 2004;39:1288–94.
17. Gottlieb A, Satariano-Hayden P, Schoenwald P, et al. The effects of carotid sinus nerve blockade on hemodynamic stability after carotid endarterectomy. J Cardiothorac Vasc Anesth 1997;11:67–71.
18. Ghosh A, Elwell C, Smith M. Review article: cerebral near-infrared spectroscopy in adults: a work in progress. Anesth Analg 2012;115:1373–83. http://dx.doi.org/10.1213/ANE.
19. Giustiniano E, Alfano A, Battistini GM, et al. Cerebral oximetry during carotid clamping: is blood pressure raising necessary? J Cardiovasc Med (Hagerstown) 2010;11(7):522–8.
20. Liu H, Giorgio A, Williams E, et al. Protocol for electrophysiological monitoring of carotid endarterectomies. J Biomed Res 2010;24(6):460–6.
21. Rockman CB, Jacobowitz GR, Lamparello PJ, et al. Immediate reexploration for the perioperative neurologic event after carotid endarterectomy: is it worthwhile? J Vasc Surg 2000;32(6):1062–70.
22. Bond R, Rerkasem K, Counsell C, et al. Routine or selective carotid artery shunting for carotid endarterectomy (and different methods of monitoring in selective shunting). Cochrane Database Syst Rev 2009;(4):CD000190.
23. AbuRahma AF, Mousa AY, Stone PA. Shunting during carotid endarterectomy. J Vasc Surg 2011;54:1502–10.
24. Howell SJ. Carotid endarterectomy. Br J Anaesth 2007;99:119–31.
25. Inoue T, Tsutsumi K, Ohwaki K, et al. Stratification of intraoperative ischemic impact by somatosensory evoked potential monitoring, diffusion-weighted imaging and magnetic resonance angiography in carotid endarterectomy with routine shunt use. Acta Neurochir (Wien) 2013;155(11):2085–96.
26. Pennekamp CW, Tromp SC, Ackerstaff RG, et al. Prediction of cerebral hyperperfusion after carotid endarterectomy with transcranial Doppler. Eur J Vasc Endovasc Surg 2012;43(4):371–6.

27. Hans SS, Jareunpoon O. Prospective evaluation of electroencephalography carotid artery stump pressure and neurologic changes during 314 consecutive carotid endarterectomies performed in awake patients. J Vasc Surg 2007;45(3): 511–5.
28. Evans WE, Hayes JP, Waltke EA, et al. Optimal cerebral monitoring during carotid endarterectomy: neurologic response under local anesthesia. J Vasc Surg 1985;2(6):775–7.
29. Ritter JC, Green D, Slim H, et al. The role of cerebral oximetry in combination with awake testing in patients undergoing carotid endarterectomy under local anaesthesia. Eur J Vasc Endovasc Surg 2011;41(5):599–605.
30. Ballotta E, Saladini M, Gruppo M, et al. Predictors of electroencephalographic changes needing shunting during carotid endarterectomy. Ann Vasc Surg 2010;24:1045–52.
31. Shang Y, Cheng R, Dong L, et al. Cerebral monitoring during carotid endarterectomy using near-infrared diffuse optical spectroscopies and electroencephalogram. Phys Med Biol 2011;56:3015.
32. Friedell ML, Clark JM, Graham DA, et al. Cerebral oximetry does not correlate with electroencephalography and somatosensory evoked potentials in determining the need for shunting during carotid endarterectomy. J Vasc Surg 2008;48:601–6.
33. Moritz S, Kasprzak P, Arlt M, et al. Accuracy of cerebral monitoring in detecting cerebral ischemia during carotid endarterectomy: a comparison of transcranial Doppler sonography, near-infrared spectroscopy, stump pressure, and somatosensory evoked potentials. Anesthesiology 2007;107:563–9.
34. Moritz S, Schmidt C, Bucher M, et al. Neuromonitoring in carotid surgery: are the results obtained in awake patients transferable to patients under sevoflurane/fentanyl anesthesia? J Neurosurg Anesthesiol 2010;22(4):288–95.
35. Guarracino F. Cerebral monitoring during cardiovascular surgery. Curr Opin Anaesthesiol 2008;21(1):50–4.
36. Foreman B, Claassen J. Quantitative EEG for the detection of brain ischemia. Crit Care 2012;16(2):216.
37. Estruch-Perez MJ, Barbera-Alacreu M, Ausina-Aguilar A, et al. Bispectral index variations in patients with neurological deficits during awake carotid endarterectomy. Eur J Anaesthesiol 2010;27:359–63.
38. Deogaonkar A, Vivar R, Bullock RE, et al. Bispectral index monitoring may not reliably indicate cerebral ischaemia during awake carotid endarterectomy. Br J Anaesth 2005;94:800–4.
39. Schneider JR, Droste JS, Schindler N, et al. Carotid endarterectomy with routine electroencephalography and selective shunting: influence of contralateral internal carotid artery occlu-sion and utility in prevention of perioperative strokes. J Vasc Surg 2003;37:239–40.
40. Allen A, Starr A, Nudleman K. Assessment of sensory function in the operating room utilizing cerebral evoked potentials: a study of fifty-six surgically anesthetized patients. Clin Neurosurg 1981;28:457–81.
41. Dinkel M, Schweiger H, Goerlitz P. Monitoring during carotid surgery: somatosensory evoked potentials vs. carotid stump pressure. J Neurosurg Anesthesiol 1992;4:167–75.
42. Fielmuth S, Uhlig T. The role of somatosensory evoked potentials in detecting cerebral ischaemia during carotid endarterectomy. Eur J Anaesthesiol 2008; 25:648–56.

43. Sbarigia E, Schioppa A, Misuraca M, et al. Somatosensory evoked potentials versus locoregional anaesthesia in the monitoring of cerebral function during carotid artery surgery: preliminary results of a prospective study. Eur J Vasc Endovasc Surg 2001;21:413–6.
44. De Vleeschauwer P, Horsch S, Matamoros R. Monitoring of somatosensory evoked potentials in carotid surgery: results, usefulness and limitations of the method. Ann Vasc Surg 1988;2:63–8.
45. Malcharek MJ, Ulkatan S, Marinò V, et al. Intraoperative monitoring of carotid endarterectomy by transcranial motor evoked potential: a multicenter study of 600 patients. Clin Neurophysiol 2013;124(5):1025–30.
46. Uchino H, Nakamura T, Kuroda S, et al. Intraoperative dual monitoring during carotid endarterectomy using motor evoked potentials and near-infrared spectroscopy. World Neurosurg 2012;78(6):651–7.
47. Moore WS, Hall AD. Carotid artery back pressure: a test of cerebral tolerance to temporary carotid occlusion. Arch Surg 1969;99(6):702–10.
48. Ricotta JJ, Charlton MH, De Weese JA. Determining criteria for shunt for shunt placement during carotid endarterectomy: EEG vs back pressur. Ann Surg 1993;198:642–5.
49. Cao P, Giordano G, Zannetti S, et al. Transcranial Doppler monitoring during carotid endarterectomy: is it appropriate for selecting patients in need of a shunt? J Vasc Surg 1997;26(6):973–80.
50. Aburahma AF, Stone PA, Hass SM, et al. Prospective randomized trial of routine versus selective shunting in carotid endarterectomy based on stump pressure. J Vasc Surg 2010;51(5):1133–8.
51. Harada RN, Comerota AJ, Good GM, et al. Stump pressure, electroencephalographic changes, and the contralateral carotid artery: another look at selective shunting. Am J Surg 1995;170:148–53.
52. Kincaid MS. Transcranial Doppler ultrasonography: a diagnostic tool of increasing utility. Curr Opin Anaesthesiol 2008;21(5):552–9.
53. Naylor AR, Sayers RD, McCarthy MJ, et al. Closing the loop: a 21-year audit of strategies for preventing stroke and death following carotid endarterectomy. Eur J Vasc Endovasc Surg 2013;46(2):161–70.
54. Pennekamp CW, Immink RV, den Ruijter HM, et al. Near-infrared spectroscopy can predict the onset of cerebral hyperperfusion syndrome after carotid endarterectomy. Cerebrovasc Dis 2012;34(4):314–21.
55. Pennekamp CW, Bots ML, Kappelle LJ, et al. The value of near-infrared spectroscopy measured cerebral oximetry during carotid endarterectomy in perioperative stroke prevention. A review. Eur J Vasc Endovasc Surg 2009;38(5):539–45.
56. Jaipersad TS, Saedon M, Tiivas C, et al. Perioperative transorbital Doppler flow imaging offers an alternative to transcranial Doppler monitoring in those patients without a temporal bone acoustic window. Ultrasound Med Biol 2011;37(5):719–22.
57. Stilo F, Spinelli F, Martelli E, et al. The sensibility and specificity of cerebral oximetry, measured by INVOS - 4100, in patients undergoing carotid endarterectomy compared with awake testing. Minerva Anestesiol 2012;78(10):1126–35.
58. Manwaring ML, Durham CA, McNally MM, et al. Correlation of cerebral oximetry with internal carotid artery stump pressures in carotid endarterectomy. Vasc Endovascular Surg 2010;44(4):252–6.
59. Tambakis CL, Papadopoulos G, Sergentanis TN, et al. Cerebral oximetry and stump pressure as indicators for shunting during carotid endarterectomy: comparative evaluation. Vascular 2011;19:187–94.

60. Mauermann WJ, Crepeau AZ, Pulido JN, et al. Comparison of electroencephalography and cerebral oximetry to determine the need for in-line arterial shunting in patients undergoing carotid endarterectomy. J Cardiothorac Vasc Anesth 2013;27(6):1253–9.
61. Pennekamp CW, Immink RV, den Ruijter HM, et al. Near-infrared spectroscopy to indicate selective shunt use during carotid endarterectomy. Eur J Vasc Endovasc Surg 2013;46(4):397–403.
62. Mille T, Tachimiri ME, Klersy C, et al. Near infrared spectroscopy monitoring during carotid endarterectomy: which threshold value is critical? Eur J Vasc Endovasc Surg 2004;27:646–50.
63. Al-Rawi PG, Kirkpatrick PJ. Tissue oxygen index: thresholds for cerebral ischemia using near-infrared spectroscopy. Stroke 2006;37:2720–5.
64. Radak D, Sotirovic V, Obradovic M, et al. Practical Use of Near-Infrared Spectroscopy in Carotid Surgery. Angiology 2013. [Epub ahead of print].
65. Guay J, Kopp S. Cerebral monitors versus regional anesthesia to detect cerebral ischemia in patients undergoing carotid endarterectomy: a meta-analysis. Can J Anaesth 2013;60(3):266–79.
66. Momin TA, Ricotta JJ. Minimizing the complications of carotid endarterectomy. Perspect Vasc Surg Endovasc Ther 2010;22(2):106–13.
67. Greenstein AJ, Chassin MR, Wang J, et al. Association between minor and major surgical complications after carotid endarterectomy: results of the New York carotid artery surgery study. J Vasc Surg 2007;46:1138–46.
68. Brott TG, Halperin JL, Abbara S, et al. 2011 ASA/ACCF/AHA/AANN/AANS/ACR/ASNR/CNS/SAIP/SCAI/SIR/SNIS/SVM/SVS guideline on the management of patients with extracranial carotid and vertebral artery disease: executive summary. A report of the American College of Cardiology Foundation/American Heart Association Task Force on Practice Guidelines, and the American Stroke Association, American Association of Neuroscience Nurses, American Association of Neurological Surgeons, American College of Radiology, American Society of Neuroradiology, Congress of Neurological Surgeons, Society of Atherosclerosis Imaging and Prevention, Society for Cardiovascular Angiography and Interventions, Society of Interventional Radiology, Society of NeuroInterventional Surgery, Society for Vascular Medicine, and Society for Vascular Surgery. Circulation 2011;124:489–532.
69. The European Carotid Surgery Trialists' Collaborative Group. Endarterectomy for moderate symptomatic carotid stenosis: interim results from the MRC European Carotid Surgery Trial. Lancet 1996;347:1591–3.
70. Heyer EJ, Adams D, Solomon RA, et al. Neuropsychometric changes in patients after carotid endarterectomy. Stroke 1998;29:1110–5.
71. Mocco J, Wilson DA, Komotar RJ, et al. Predictors of neurocognitive decline after carotid endarterectomy. Neurosurgery 2006;58:844–50.
72. Rockman CB, Su W, Lamparello PJ, et al. A reassessment of carotid endarterectomy in the face of contralateral carotid occlusion: surgical results in symptomatic and asymptomatic patients. J Vasc Surg 2002;36(4):668–73.
73. Fassiadis N, Zayed H, Rashid H, et al. Invos Cerebral Oximeter compared with the transcranial Doppler for monitoring adequacy of cerebral perfusion in patients undergoing carotid endarterectomy. Int Angiol 2006;25:401–6.
74. Hertzer NR, Young JR, Beven EG, et al. Coronary angiography in 506 patients with extracranial cerebrovascular disease. Arch Intern Med 1985;145(5):849–52.
75. North American Symptomatic Carotid Endarterectomy Trial Collaborators. Beneficial effect of carotid endarterectomy in symp-tomatic patients with high-grade carotid stenosis. N Engl J Med 1991;325:445–53.

76. Aksoy O, Kapadia SR, Bajzer C, et al. Carotid stenting vs surgery: parsing the risk of stroke and MI. Cleve Clin J Med 2010;77(12):892–902.
77. Blackshear JL, Brott TG. Ascertainment of any and all neurologic and myocardial damage in carotid revascularization: the key to optimization? Expert Rev Cardiovasc Ther 2013;11(4):469–84.
78. Stoneham MD, Thompson JP. Arterial pressure management and carotid endarterectomy. Br J Anaesth 2009;102(4):442–52.
79. van Mook WN, Rennenberg RJ, Schurink GW, et al. Cerebral hyperperfusion syndrome. Lancet Neurol 2005;4(12):877–88.
80. Pennekamp CW, Moll FL, De Borst GJ. Role of transcranial Doppler in cerebral hyperperfusion syndrome. J Cardiovasc Surg (Torino) 2012;53(6):765–71.
81. Ogasawara K, Sakai N, Kuroiwa T, et al. Intracranial hemorrhage associated with cerebral hyperperfusion syndrome following carotid endarterectomy and carotid artery stenting: retrospective review of 4494 patients. J Neurosurg 2007;107:1130–6.
82. Komoribayashi N, Ogasawara K, Kobayashi M, et al. Cerebral hyperperfusion after carotid endarterectomy is associated with preoperative hemodynamic impairment and intraoperative cerebral ischemia. J Cereb Blood Flow Metab 2006;26:878–84.
83. Liu B, Lai ZC, Ni L, et al. New method to predict cerebral hyperperfusion syndrome after carotid endarterectomy by transcranial Doppler. Zhonghua Wai Ke Za Zhi 2013;51(6):504–7.
84. Ogasawara K, Konno H, Yukawa H, et al. Transcranial regional cerebral oxygen saturation monitoring during carotid endarterectomy as a predictor of postoperative hyperperfusion. Neurosurgery 2003;53(2):309–14 [discussion: 314–5].
85. Erickson KM, Cole DJ. Carotid artery disease: stenting vs endarterectomy. Br J Anaesth 2010;105(Suppl 1):i34–49.
86. Abbott AL. Medical (nonsurgical) intervention alone is now best for prevention of stroke associated with asymptomatic severe carotid stenosis: results of a systematic review and analysis. Stroke 2009;13:e573–83.

Perioperative Management of Combined Carotid and Coronary Artery Bypass Grafting Procedures

Daryl A. Oakes, MD*, Kenneth D. Eichenbaum, MD, MSE

KEYWORDS

- Staged carotid and coronary artery bypass graft surgery
- Combined carotid and coronary artery bypass graft surgery
- Perioperative anesthetic management • Carotid artery stenosis
- Carotid artery stenting • Carotid endarterectomy

KEY POINTS

- Perioperative stroke is most commonly secondary to embolic phenomena, but multiple causes can be involved.
- Current data show no clear difference in complication rates for stroke, myocardial infarction, and death between staged versus combined carotid and coronary artery bypass graft (CABG) repairs, though prospective controlled studies are needed.
- Given the generally higher rates of neurologic sequelae with combined carotid/CABG procedures (staged or simultaneous), combined repair is generally performed in patients with both severe coronary artery disease and symptomatic or severe carotid disease.
- Anesthetic and perioperative management should be focused on minimizing the risk for perioperative complications, especially stroke and myocardial infarction.

INTRODUCTION

The efficient diagnostic and therapeutic management of patients with concurrent carotid and coronary disease presents a significant clinical challenge. The avoidance of devastating complications of stroke, myocardial infarction (MI) and death,[1] particularly within 30 days[2] of surgical intervention, is a primary goal. A review of the morbidity and mortality of various surgical management options in this problematic

Funding Sources: None.
Conflict of Interest: None.
Division of Cardiothoracic Anesthesia, Department of Anesthesiology, Perioperative and Pain Medicine, Stanford University Medical Center, 300 Pasteur Drive H3580, MC 5640, Stanford, CA 94305, USA
* Corresponding author.
E-mail address: doakes@stanford.edu

Anesthesiology Clin 32 (2014) 699–721
http://dx.doi.org/10.1016/j.anclin.2014.05.005 **anesthesiology.theclinics.com**
1932-2275/14/$ – see front matter

patient population can facilitate a more systematic clinical approach to perioperative management strategies.

PERIOPERATIVE STROKE RISK IN CORONARY ARTERY BYPASS GRAFT

Overall, postoperative stroke complicates 1% to 2% of all isolated coronary artery bypass graft (CABG) surgery and can confer a 3- to 6-fold increased risk of mortality.[3–6] Carotid artery stenosis has been recognized as a significant risk factor for perioperative stroke in this population. As a result, strategies to identify and actively manage significant carotid artery disease before CABG have been developed, including carotid revascularization contemporaneously with coronary surgery. There is significant debate over which surgical strategies in this patient population are the most effective.

Irrespective of carotid artery disease, the overall stroke rates after isolated CABG surgery have declined over the last several decades (**Fig. 1**).[7,8] This improvement is likely to be caused, in part, by improved medical therapy for cerebrovascular disease (eg, antiplatelet therapy, statin therapy, aggressive management of hypertension). Additionally, significant improvements in perioperative management have occurred, including efforts to minimize aortic manipulation, the implementation of arterial line filters and membrane oxygenators in the cardiopulmonary bypass circuit, efforts to optimize cerebral perfusion, careful intraoperative control of metabolic derangements and hyperglycemia, and postoperative management of cardiac dysrhythmias.

Although stroke continues to be a significant source of perioperative morbidity, this trend of improvement suggests a powerful opportunity for the perioperative physician to positively impact outcomes in these patients independent of the surgical strategy used. An in-depth understanding of the best diagnostic and perioperative options is important for optimizing management and improving outcomes. As a care provider, it is, therefore, incumbent to understand the best practices for the management of these complex patients.

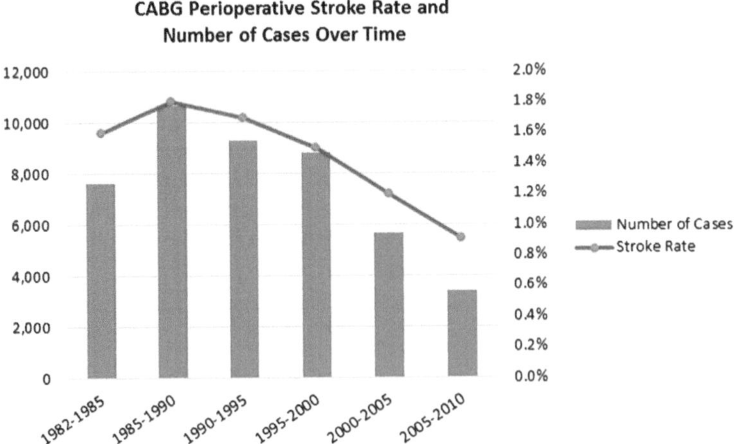

Fig. 1. Rate of stroke after CABG over last several decades. A major study of 45,432 patients at the Cleveland Clinic from 1982 to 2009 demonstrated the decline of perioperative stroke after CABG surgery. (*Data from* Tarakji KG, Sabik JF, Bhudia SK, et al. Temporal onset, risk factors, and outcomes associated with stroke after coronary artery bypass grafting. JAMA 2011;305(4):381–90.)

Cause of Perioperative Stroke After CABG

To date, the mechanisms of perioperative stroke after CABG have been poorly elucidated. The available data suggest that most perioperative strokes seem to be embolic in nature, either resulting from intracardiac thrombi (cardioembolic) or atherosclerotic disease of the carotid artery, the aortic arch, or the ascending aorta.[9] Additionally, emboli can be generated from debris or air entrained from the surgical field. Although less common, other stroke causes may also play a role (**Fig. 2**).

Strokes classified as ischemic in nature include thrombotic strokes resulting from acute plaque rupture or hypercoagulability; lacunar strokes, which are small areas of ischemic injury resulting from chronic hypertension and associated atherosclerotic and stenotic lesions in small vessels of the deep cerebral white matter; and hypoperfusion or watershed strokes, which are associated with systemic hypotension. Hemorrhagic stroke is less common in the setting of CABG and is associated with extravasation of blood resulting cerebral edema, tissue compression, and injury. Recognizing the mechanisms underlying perioperative stroke is fundamental to decreasing the incidence of major neurologic events. Given our inability to predict specific events in individual patients, and the fact that a significant number of strokes seem to have multiple causes, a multifaceted approach to prevention seems warranted.[9–11]

Risk Factors for Perioperative Stroke with CABG

The rate of stroke has been demonstrated to increase with age: risk of stroke at 50 years of age is 0.5%, and at 80 years of age it is greater than 8.0%.[5,12–14] Besides age, multiple risk factors have been identified as being independently predictive of perioperative stroke after CABG (**Table 1**).

The identified risk factors are listed in **Table 1**. Additionally, several intraoperative and postoperative factors have also been identified to be independent predictors of perioperative stroke. Important contributors to increased neurologic morbidity include prolonged cardiopulmonary bypass times, manipulation of atherosclerotic aorta,

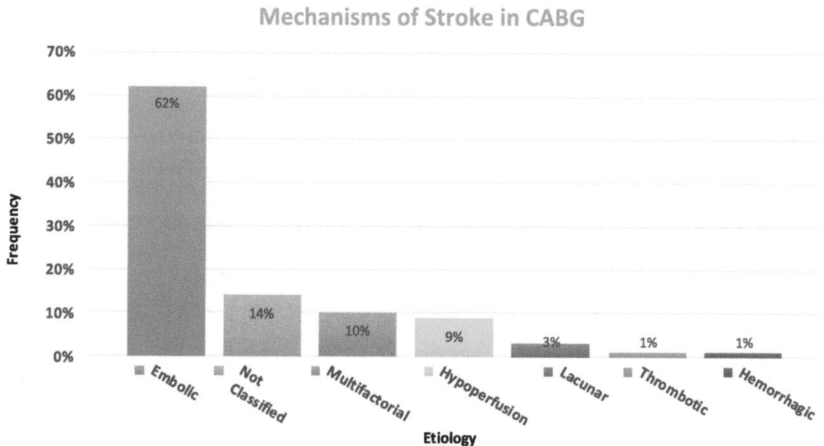

Fig. 2. Stroke causes. Although most perioperative strokes are a result of embolic origin, several other stroke mechanisms may occur. (*Data from* Likosky DS, Marrin CA, Caplan LR, et al. Determination of etiologic mechanisms of strokes secondary to coronary artery bypass graft surgery. Stroke 2003;34(12):2830–4.)

Table 1
Risk factors for perioperative stroke after CABG

Patient Factors	Preoperative	Intraoperative	Postoperative
Advanced age Neurologic, carotid, valvular, pulmonary or peripheral vascular disease Dysrhythmia CABG or MI Unstable angina Congestive heart failure Heavy alcohol intake Hypertension	Systolic BP >180 mm Hg Antihypertensive therapy	Proximal aortic atherosclerosis Intraoperative hypotension Aortic balloon pump Use of atrial or ventricular vent	Dysrhythmia Congestive heart failure

Abbreviation: BP, blood pressure.

Data from Roach GW, Kanchuger M, Mangano CM, et al. Adverse cerebral outcomes after coronary bypass surgery. N Engl J Med 1996;335(25):1857–64; and Merie C, Kober L, Olsen PS, et al. Risk of stroke after coronary artery bypass grafting: effect of age and comorbidities. Stroke 2012;43(1):38–43.

hypotension, low cardiac output syndrome, intra-aortic balloon pumps, and postoperative atrial fibrillation.[5,12]

Carotid Disease and Perioperative Stroke Risk with CABG

Strategies for combined carotid and coronary revascularization have been developed to address the increased risk of perioperative stroke associated with moderate to severe carotid stenosis in patients undergoing CABG. A review of the Society of Thoracic Surgery's database from 2003 to 2007 suggested that the presence of cerebrovascular disease increases the risk of stroke to 2.72% in comparison with 1.0% in patients without cerebrovascular disease.[3] Increasing carotid disease burden seems to be associated with a higher risk of stroke after CABG. In a systematic review by Naylor and colleagues,[6] the rate of stroke increased from 1.8% in CABG patients without carotid disease to 3.0% with unilateral stenosis (50%–99%), 5% with bilateral stenosis (50%–99%), and 7% to 11% in patients with carotid occlusion (**Fig. 3**).

Symptomatic patients, those with a history of stroke or transient ischemic attack (TIA), seem to be at the highest risk. In the noncardiac surgical population, symptomatic patients with 50% or more carotid stenosis who do not undergo carotid revascularization have a 3-month recurrent stroke rate of 32%.[15] In the setting of CABG, a history of TIA or stroke has been associated with a 4-fold increase in perioperative stroke.[16] The risk of postoperative stroke after CABG in patients with symptomatic carotid disease has been reported to be 18% for those with unilateral carotid stenosis and as high as 26% for bilateral stenosis.[13]

Screening for Carotid Disease

Approximately 9% to 22% of CABG patients[6,17–19] have significant carotid disease (>50% stenosis). Severe carotid stenosis (>80%) is found in 8% to 12% of patients presenting for CABG (**Fig. 4**).[17] The relatively high prevalence of carotid disease in the CABG population, and its association with an elevated risk of perioperative stroke, has led to more aggressive efforts to identify patients with concomitant carotid and coronary disease preoperatively.

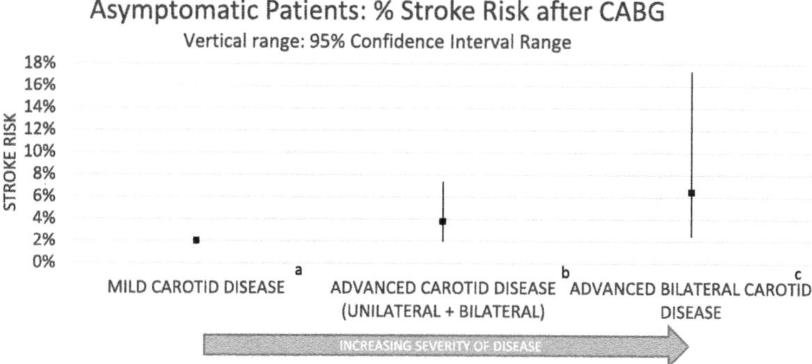

Fig. 3. Plot of stroke risks in asymptomatic patients with progressively advanced carotid disease. [a] MILD CAROTID DISEASE: carotid stenosis less than 50% (n = 7685).[4] [b] ADVANCED CAROTID DISEASE: encompasses patients with 50% to 99% unilateral, 50% to 99% unilateral with contralateral occlusion, or 50% to 99% bilateral stenoses. No prior neurologic events (n = 931).[6] [c] ADVANCED BILATERAL CAROTID DISEASE: 50% to 99% bilateral or 50% to 99% unilateral + contralateral occlusion (n = 206).[6] (*Data from* Naylor AR, Mehta Z, Rothwell PM, et al. Carotid artery disease and stroke during coronary artery bypass: a critical review of the literature. Eur J Vasc Endovasc Surg 2002;23(4):283–94; and Naylor AR, Bown MJ. Stroke after cardiac surgery and its association with asymptomatic carotid disease: an updated systematic review and meta-analysis. Eur J Vasc Endovasc Surg 2011;41(5):607–24.)

Although many centers have implemented universal carotid imaging to screen for carotid disease in all CABG patients, more recently, many studies have suggested that this approach is not necessary. Carotid stenosis seems to be associated with specific patient characteristics.[19–21] Patients with these high-risk characteristics have a significantly greater prevalence of disease than the low-risk population, 17.8% versus 6.1%, respectively.[19] Given this association, the 2011 American College of Cardiology Foundation/American Heart Association's (ACCF/AHA) guidelines recommends that "carotid artery duplex scanning is reasonable in selected patients who are considered to have high-risk features (ie, age >65 years, left main coronary stenosis, peripheral artery disease, history of cerebrovascular disease [transient ischemic attack, stroke, etc.], hypertension, smoking, and diabetes mellitus). (Class IIa, Level of Evidence: C)."[22] (**Box 1**, **Fig. 5**).

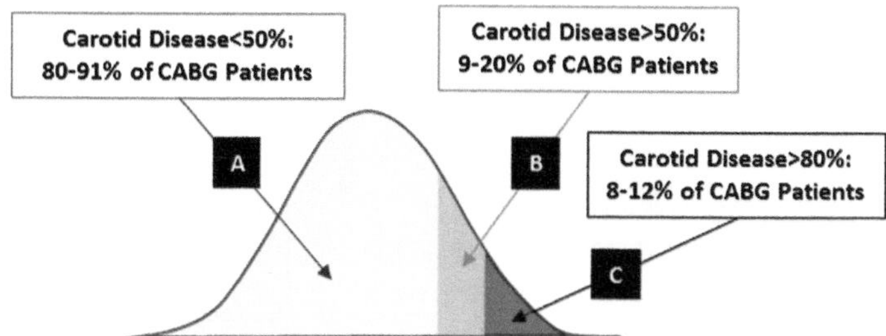

Fig. 4. Prevalence of carotid disease in the CABG population. (*A*) Mild carotid disease is present in up to 91% of CABG patients. (*B*) Patients with carotid stenosis greater than 50% compose approximately 9% to 20% of CABG patients (*Blue and Red shaded area*). (*C*) Severe carotid disease is present in 8% to 12% of CABG patients. (*Data from* Refs.[6,18])

Box 1
The ACC/AHA's recommendations for screening with carotid duplex

- Age greater than 65 years
- Left main coronary stenosis
- Peripheral artery disease
- Smokers
- Prior TIA/stroke
- Active carotid bruit

Carotid Disease as a Marker of Risk Versus Source of Morbidity

Although carotid disease is clearly associated with increased risk of stroke after CABG, surgical carotid intervention may not fully address the problem. It has been argued that the cause of perioperative stroke may relate to pervasive atheromatous disease rather than primarily disease of the carotid vessels. No significant carotid stenosis is detected in 50% to 75% of perioperative strokes after CABG.[6,23] Lee and colleagues[24] suggest that intracranial and noncarotid, extracranial atherosclerotic disease rather than carotid disease is predictive of stroke. They reviewed 1367 consecutive CABG patients who underwent preoperative and postoperative cerebral

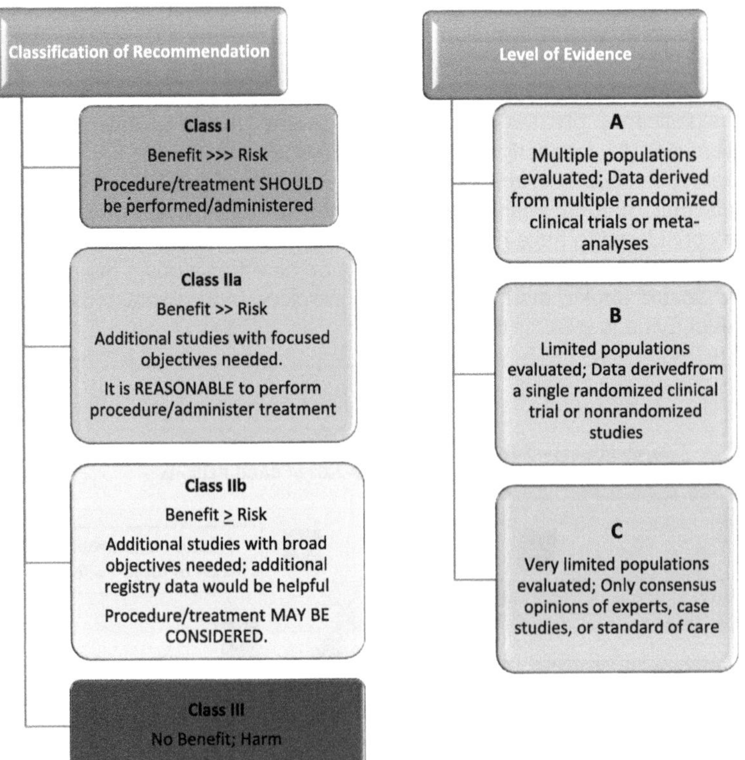

Fig. 5. Classification of recommendations and levels of evidence.

magnetic resonance angiography. Of the 33 patients who had a stroke, 15 had strokes characterized as atherosclerotic in origin; only 7 of these individuals had carotid artery disease. Of these 7 patients, only 3 patients had strokes that could be attributed to the carotid lesion.[24] Additionally, as noted earlier, a significant percentage of perioperative strokes after CABG are multifactorial in origin,[8,9] making carotid disease only one of several important factors to modify (**Box 2**).

SURGICAL TREATMENT STRATEGIES

Options for Intervention

The surgical management options for patients with both significant carotid and coronary disease have traditionally been either a staged approach with initial carotid endarterectomy followed by CABG as a second procedure at a later time point versus a simultaneous procedure in which carotid and coronary revascularization occur in one operative setting. During simultaneous revascularization, carotid endarterectomy (CEA) may be performed either before bypass, during harvesting of the left internal mammary graft, or during cardiopulmonary bypass (CPB). The cervical wound is usually left open and packed until after separation from CPB and protamine administration. More recently, endovascular carotid artery stenting (CAS) has become a potential alternative to open carotid surgery in these patients (see **Fig. 5**). Additionally, although less common, staged procedures may be timed such that the CEA is performed as a separate surgery after CABG, referred to as *reverse staged* procedures.

Overall Complication Rates by Type of Intervention

The appropriate surgical treatment option to address simultaneous carotid and coronary disease is the subject of a significant amount of debate in the surgical literature. The data currently available are from retrospective reports and meta-analyses, but there are no prospective controlled trials that directly compare the relative safety and efficacy of each approach in specific patient populations. Although a complete review of the discussion is beyond the scope of this article, the authors briefly summarize the issues associated with each therapeutic approach here.

In a systematic review of 94 separate studies published in 2003, simultaneous CEA/CABG was associated with a risk of death, stroke, or MI of 11.5% (95% confidence interval [CI] 10.1–12.9) compared with 10.2% (95% CI 7.4–13.1) for staged CEA then CABG.[2] Although the risk of stroke and/or death was higher with simultaneous compared with staged repair (8.7%, 95% CI 7.7–9.8; vs 6.1%, 95% CI 2.9–9.3), MI was more frequent with staged procedures (6.5%, 95% CI 3.2–9.7 vs combined 3.6%, 95% CI 3.0–4.2) (**Fig. 6**).[2]

Box 2
Important facts

- The estimated incidence of stroke is 1% to 2% in CABG patients without cardiovascular disease.
- This rate increases to 2.72% in patients with cerebrovascular disease undergoing CABG.
- The presence of significant bilateral carotid disease or symptomatic carotid disease is associated with increased risk of perioperative stroke after CABG.
- Perioperative stroke after CABG is most frequently caused by embolic phenomena.
- Carotid disease may be a marker for stroke risk rather than a cause of morbidity.

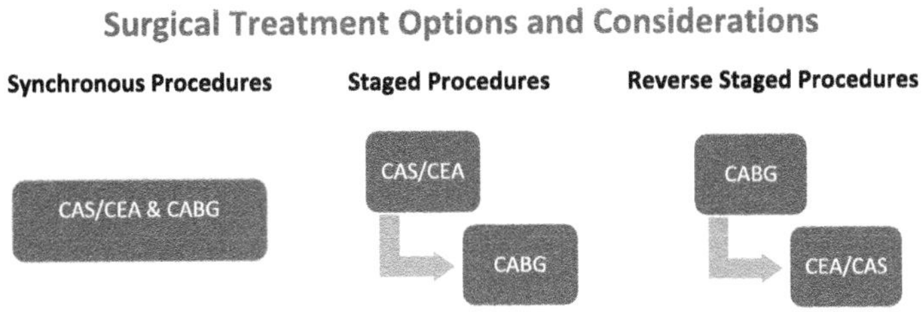

Surgical Treatment Options and Considerations

Synchronous Procedures — CAS/CEA & CABG

Staged Procedures — CAS/CEA → CABG

Reverse Staged Procedures — CABG → CEA/CAS

Fig. 6. Options for Intervention. In patients with combined carotid and vascular disease, the procedures are generally performed in 3 distinct ways: synchronous, staged, and reverse staged.

Similarly, several other studies have also shown that when CEA is performed before coronary revascularization, there were fewer stroke complications but increases in the numbers of MI.[6,21,25] On the other hand, reverse staged procedures (ie, CABG is performed before carotid revascularization) were associated with the lowest MI rate (0.9%, 95% CI 0.5–1.4); however, the stroke rate (6.3%, 95% CI 1.0–11.7) was higher than observed in the other surgical approaches.[2]

A 2012 systematic review of combined carotid-coronary procedures by Venkatachalam and colleagues[26] reported early outcomes as follows: combined CEA/CABG: stroke 4% (0%–18%, n = 10,243), MI 3% (0%–13%, n = 7027), and death 5% (0%–14%, n = 11,854); staged CEA/CABG: stroke 2% (0%–8%, n = 933), MI 6% (0%–29%, n = 933), and death 4% (0%–33%, n = 919); and reverse staged procedures: stroke 5% (0%–14%, n = 335), MI 1% (0%–5%, n = 335), and death 3% (0%–13%, n = 335). Gopaldas and colleagues[27] reviewed the Nationwide Inpatient Sample database from 1998 to 2007 for results of staged prior or subsequent CEA with CABG (n = 6153) versus combined CEA/CABG (n = 16,639) and found no significant difference in neurologic and mortality outcomes. They did note a higher morbidity (48.4% vs 42.6%; odds ratio1.8, 95% CI 1.5–2.2) and increased hospital costs ($23,328; *P*<.001) for staged procedures.[27]

Patient Selection for Combined or Staged Procedures

Given that the goal of carotid revascularization in the setting of cardiac surgery is to reduce the risk of procedural-related stroke, generally only patient populations at the highest risk for a perioperative stroke with CABG are considered for combined or staged carotid-coronary procedures. According to the ACCF/AHA's 2011 guidelines, these patients include those with symptomatic carotid stenosis of 50% to 99% (class IIa, evidence C), patients with bilateral asymptomatic stenosis of 80% to 99%, or unilateral carotid stenosis of 70% to 99% with contralateral occlusion (class IIb, evidence C) (**Fig. 7**).[8,17,18,22,25] Patients with asymptomatic unilateral carotid stenosis of 50% to 99% with no history of stroke seem to have a low risk of perioperative stroke. As a result, some investigators suggest that these patients' carotid disease may be best managed medically (**Box 3**, **Fig. 8**).[28]

Currently, there is little definitive evidence to guide decision making with regard to procedure timing, that is, whether to perform carotid revascularization as part of a combined procedure versus manage it as 2 separate, staged interventions. Although procedural timing is controversial and varies by institution, in general, in clinical practice, the acuity of the respective lesions guides decision making. The more symptomatic lesion (carotid or coronary) is frequently addressed first in a staged procedure; however, depending on the experience of the particular institution, revascularization may be performed in a combined procedure performed in one anesthetic.[27] For

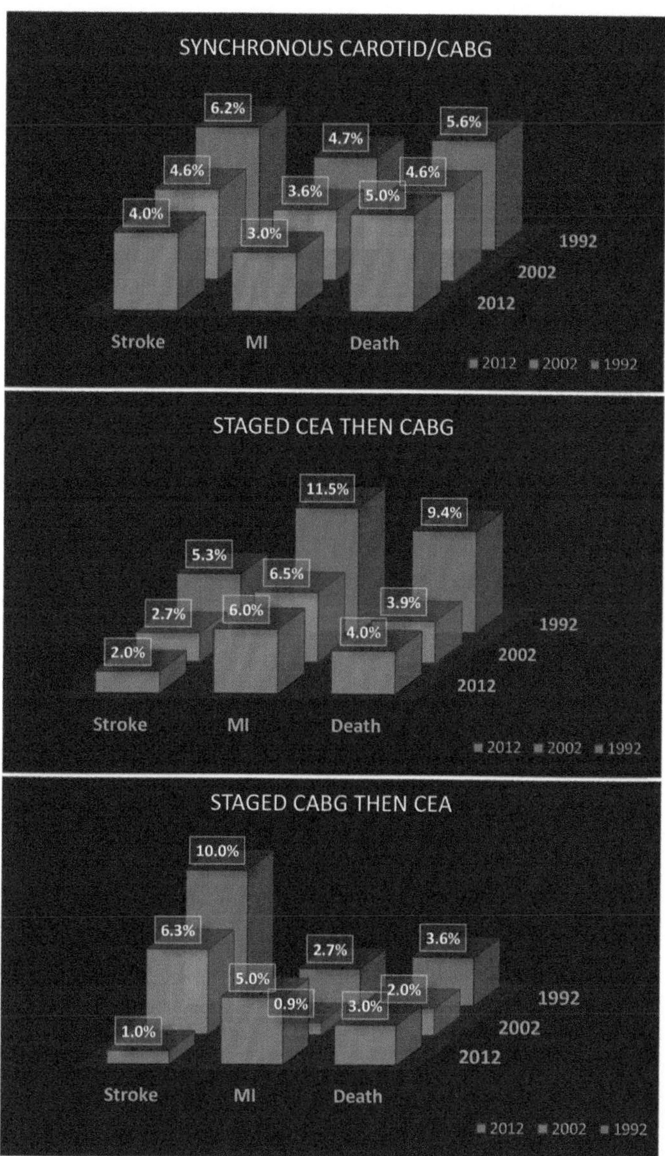

Fig. 7. Complication rates of stroke, MI, and death over 3 decades for staged and synchronous carotid/CABG surgeries. (*Data from* Naylor AR, Mehta Z, Rothwell PM, et al. Carotid artery disease and stroke during coronary artery bypass: a critical review of the literature. Eur J Vasc Endovasc Surg 2002;23(4):283–94; and Venkatachalam S, Gray BH, Shishehbor MH. Open and endovascular management of concomitant severe carotid and coronary artery disease: tabular review of the literature. Ann Vasc Surg 2012;26(1):125–40.)

patients with symptomatic carotid disease and active coronary lesions (eg, severe left main disease or unstable angina), many institutions would favor simultaneous repair with CEA/CABG.[13,27,29] Whether carotid stenting should be considered in this setting is yet another area of debate (see "Method of carotid revascularization" section). Additionally, no consensus exists for how to time revascularization for patients with more

Box 3
Guidelines for medical treatment for asymptomatic carotid disease

- Treat hypertensive patients with antihypertensives to goal a blood pressure of less than 140/90 (class I, evidence: A).
- Encourage smoking cessation with interventions to reduce atherosclerosis and stroke (class I, evidence: B).
- Target low-density lipoprotein (LDL) cholesterol less than 100 mg/dL with statins (class I, evidence: B) (and less than 70 mg/dL in patients with diabetes mellitus [class IIa, evidence: B]).
- If statins do not achieve the target goals, use additional LDL lowering agents (eg, niacin or bile acid sequestrants) (class IIa, evidence: B).
- Take aspirin, 75 to 325 mg, daily for extracranial atherosclerosis (class I, evidence: A).
- Take clopidogrel or ticlopidine if aspirin is contraindicated (class IIa, evidence: C).

stable coronary lesions (eg, chronic stable angina) who present with concurrent, severe carotid disease (symptomatic or asymptomatic); these patients are variously managed with staged procedures or simultaneous revascularization.

METHOD OF CAROTID REVASCULARIZATION

Limited data are available to help distinguish which patients should be selected for open carotid intervention (CEA) versus endovascular carotid stent grafting (CAS). Although studies comparing CAS and CEA in patients with isolated carotid disease

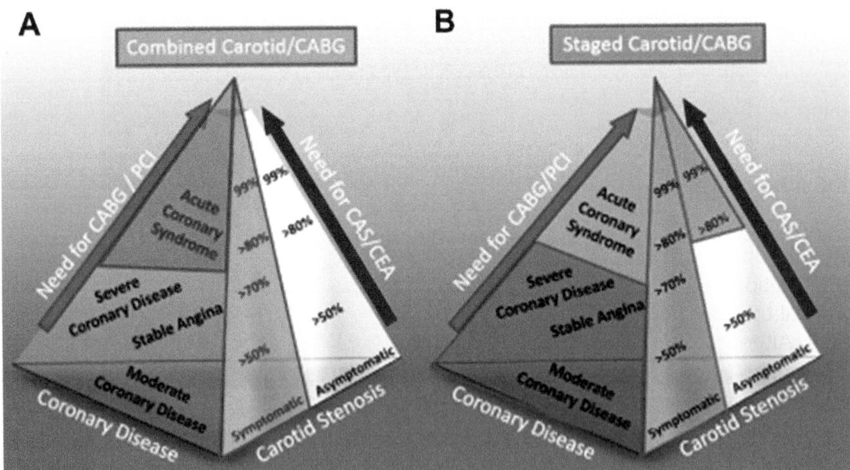

Fig. 8. Decision-making for combined and staged carotid/CABG repair. The decision to perform combined versus staged carotid/CABG can be visualized in the decision matrix shown. The arrows show increasing need for CABG/Percutaneous Intervention (*red arrow*) and increasing need for CAS/CEA (*blue arrow*) as the severity of presentation increases. (*A*) Combined carotid/ CABG surgery may be favored when there is urgent/emergent need for coronary vascularization in the setting of severe, symptomatic carotid disease (*red shaded area*). (*B*) Staged carotid/CABG surgery are a reasonable option when the CABG is non-urgent need for CABG and the patients are either symptomatic with carotid stenosis exceeding 50% or they are asymptomatic with high-grade stenosis (*gray shaded area*).

(ie, no concurrent need for CABG) have suggested that both approaches have good long-term outcomes,[30] it seems that the periprocedural risk of stroke may be higher in patients undergoing CAS. The periprocedural risk seems to be higher in elderly patients (>70 years of age) and symptomatic patients undergoing CAS as compared with CEA.[31,32] In all groups, however, isolated CEA, is associated with a higher rate of perioperative MI.[33] In a systematic review designed to evaluate CAS before CABG, Guzman and colleagues[34] pooled 6 retrospective studies and found 277 patients having staged carotid artery stents placed followed by CABG. They reported a 4.7% incidence of stroke and death following stenting and a 2.2% stroke rate related to CABG. The overall incidence of death and any associated strokes was 12.3%.

As a result, there is no clear evidence to guide the choice of CEA versus CAS for carotid revascularization in patients with concurrent severe coronary disease. Decision making can be affected by the need for aggressive antiplatelet therapy after CAS. In studies of patients undergoing simultaneous CAS/CABG, antiplatelet therapy was started 6 to 10 hours postoperatively; but increased rates of perioperative bleeding complications were observed.[35] As a result, CAS is frequently used as part of a staged procedure with 4 weeks of antiplatelet therapy following stent placement and before CABG. In the setting of unfavorable surgical access (eg, high bifurcation of the carotid, history of neck radiation, or prior CEA), CAS may be preferred. CAS in these settings is a class IIa, evidence B recommendation in the ACCF/AHA's 2011 guidelines for carotid and vascular disease.

PERIOPERATIVE MANAGEMENT

Anesthetic Considerations

Regardless of surgical timing or approach, this patient population, presenting with severe disease in both carotid and coronary vascular beds, is at high risk for perioperative complications, particularly stroke. As a result, anesthesia providers seeking to optimize outcomes in the combined carotid/CABG population need to address several concerns. These concerns include preoperative optimization, monitoring and preservation of cerebral oxygenation in the perioperative period, and interventions for circumstances of hemodynamic derangement.

Preoperative Management

Medical optimization

Patient populations presenting with concomitant carotid and coronary disease have, by definition, advanced atherosclerotic disease burden. When possible, optimizing medical therapy for these patients can help reduce perioperative morbidity and mortality. Although data on perioperative medical therapy specific to patients with concomitant disease are limited, the extensive evidence amassed in noncardiac, vascular patients and patients undergoing isolated coronary artery surgery can be informative. In patients with a significant risk of perioperative stroke and MI, mainstays of medical preventative therapy include smoking cessation, control of hypertension and diabetes mellitus, antiplatelet therapy, and statin therapy to lower serum lipid.[36,37]

Control of hypertension

Patients with poorly controlled hypertension are intravascularly depleted and frequently demonstrate increased intraoperative hemodynamic lability. Hypertension has long been recognized as a risk factor for perioperative stroke in coronary artery bypass surgery.[12] Even in the general (nonsurgical) population, hypertension has been associated with an increased risk of stroke. Each 6- to 5-mm Hg decrease in systolic blood pressure decreases the risk of stroke by 38%,[38] and adequate blood pressure management (<140/90) is recommended by the ASA/ACCF/AHA's guidelines for asymptomatic carotid stenosis (class I, evidence A).[21]

In the setting of *symptomatic* carotid disease, however, the best practice for blood pressure management is unclear. For patients with symptomatic disease, given the risk of hypoperfusion secondary to low blood pressures, no systolic blood pressure goals have been established. Additionally, patients who have had an acute stroke demonstrate impaired cerebral vascular autoregulation, making them more susceptible to cerebral injury in the setting of decreased blood pressures. As a result, although control of hypertension is generally a priority in patients with coronary or cerebral vascular disease, careful consideration is necessary when managing hypertension in symptomatic patients undergoing combined carotid-coronary revascularization.

Beta-blocker therapy

The role of beta-blocker therapy in this population is currently poorly defined. In patients undergoing isolated coronary surgery, beta-blocker therapy seems to decrease mortality and the risk of atrial fibrillation (itself associated with postprocedural stroke). Additionally, acute withdrawal of beta-blockade has been associated with an increased risk of atrial fibrillation. The current guidelines from the ACCF/AHA for the management of isolated coronary bypass surgery patients, recommend beta-blockers be used greater than 24 hours before CABG (class I, evidence B), right after CABG (class I, evidence B), and at discharge (class I, evidence C) for all noncontraindicated patients to decrease chances for atrial fibrillation.[22] Beta-blockers may confer a mortality benefit for noncontraindicated patients with left ventricular ejection fraction greater than 30%, and they may reduce perioperative myocardial ischemia (class IIa, evidence B).[22]

However, there is currently much concern about the use of beta-blocker therapy in patients undergoing noncoronary or major vascular surgery. The perioperative ischemia evaluation study (POISE) trial evaluated extended-release metoprolol on beta-blockade in a large randomized trial of non–cardiac surgery patients; although they reported a 30% decrease in nonfatal MI, there was a 33% (3.1% vs 2.3%) increase in mortality and twice the stroke rate (1.0% vs 0.5%).[39] Therefore, in patients undergoing combined carotid-coronary revascularization, the reduced risk of atrial fibrillation (and the associated risk of stroke) offered by beta-blocker therapy must be weighed against the apparent risk of cerebral injury from hyperperfusion (caused by decreased cardiac output and hypotension).

Angiotensin-converting enzyme inhibitors

Angiotensin-converting enzyme inhibitors (ACE-I) have become an integral part of hypertensive therapy, particularly in the diabetic population with renal disease. No clear evidence of benefit has been demonstrated for the use of these agents in the immediate perioperative period. Given the association with ACE-I and refractory hypotension after the induction of general anesthesia, these agents are generally held the day of surgery.

Statin therapy

Extensive data have accumulated to suggest that 3-hydroxy-3-methylglutaryl coenzyme A reductase inhibitors (statins) can have a powerful role in stabilizing atherosclerotic plaques and decreasing morbidity of atherosclerotic disease.[21] Studies in isolated CEA have demonstrated that perioperative statin therapy is associated with decreased perioperative stroke and decreased mortality.[40–42] A meta-analysis of 30,000 cardiac surgical patients found that statin therapy was associated with significant decreases in perioperative stroke and mortality.[43] The antiinflammatory effects of statins are also correlated with decreased rates of ischemic stroke and are associated with a decreased risk of perioperative atrial fibrillation.[30] Therefore, unless contraindicated, perioperative statin therapy is highly recommended (class I, evidence A) to decrease the risk of stroke and should be strongly considered in the high-risk populations undergoing carotid surgery, coronary surgery, or combined carotid-coronary revascularization.

Antiplatelet therapy

Aspirin irreversibly inhibits cyclooxygenase 1 and 2 and is thought to play a role in stabilizing atherosclerotic plaques, improving myocardial oxygen supply and demand relationships, and decreasing thrombotic and systemic inflammatory responses to surgery.[44] The combination of aspirin, beta-blocker, and statin therapy in the context of major vascular surgery has been associated with a 3-fold decrease in MI and an 8-fold decrease in 12-month mortality.[44] In the setting of CABG, aspirin has also been shown to decrease saphenous vein graft thrombosis, mortality, MI, stroke, and renal failure.[45,46] An increased risk of significant bleeding complications has not been shown to be associated with perioperative aspirin use. The ACCF/AHA's 2011 recommendations call for aspirin administration in CABG patients preoperatively (class 1, evidence B) as well as postoperatively within 6 hours (class 1, evidence A).[22]

Newer platelet inhibitors, namely, $P2Y_{12}$ receptor inhibitors (eg, clopidogrel, prasugrel, ticagrelor) and glycoprotein IIb to IIIa receptor inhibitors (eg, abciximab, eptifibatide, tirofiban), have powerful antiplatelet effects and play an important role in the management of acute coronary syndromes and acute ischemic stroke. They are used prophylactically to prevent thrombosis of coronary and carotid stent grafts. Given the risks of perioperative bleeding complications, the ACCF/AHA's 2011 guidelines recommend withdrawing these medications preoperatively. When possible, clopidogrel and ticagrelor should be stopped at least 5 days before CABG surgery (class I, evidence B) and prasugrel at least 7 days prior (class I, evidence C). Eptifibatide and tirofiban therapy should be stopped 2 to 4 hours in advance and abciximab 12 hours (class I, evidence B). In the setting of urgent surgery after recent stent placement (<4 weeks), however, $P2Y_{12}$ receptor inhibitors may need to be continued to prevent stent graft thrombosis in the perioperative period.[22,47,48]

Intraoperative Management

Although limited data exist to support specific anesthesia techniques in this population, anesthetic management can be guided by basic principles that address the specific risk factors of this particular patient population. Given the nature of combined CEA/CABG, general anesthesia with endotracheal intubation is generally required. For staged procedures, in which isolated CEA is performed in a separate anesthetic before CABG, regional anesthesia may be an option for carotid revascularization, though no data exist to support a regional technique over general anesthesia in these patients. In the setting of general anesthesia, several studies reported no change in CABG outcomes based on anesthetics used.[49,50] For maintenance of anesthesia, volatile anesthetics are often blended with short-acting hypnotics and opioids, which lack negative inotropy in most clinical doses and help fast track postoperative care. Although many anesthetic techniques can achieve acceptable results in this patient population, attention to physiologic and pathophysiologic principles is tantamount.

Hemodynamic management goals

Careful hemodynamic management including the avoidance of the extremes of heart rate (ie, avoidance of significant tachycardia or bradycardia) and blood pressure (ie, severe hypertension or hypotension) is a priority. Induction of anesthesia requires particular attention to these parameters and can be achieved with several techniques, including but not limited to narcotic-based inductions or careful titration of hypnotic agents, such as propofol or etomidate. The availability of medications, such as alpha-receptor agonists (eg, phenylephrine) and short-acting beta-receptor blockers (eg, esmolol), can also be helpful in addressing acute hemodynamic derangements. Agents with significant beta-agonist effects (eg, ephedrine and epinephrine) should be used cautiously given their potential to increase myocardial oxygen demand and myocardial ischemia.

Preinduction placement of invasive monitoring, such as arterial blood pressure monitoring, is highly recommended to allow for tight control of blood pressure during this period. Preinduction placement of central access and monitoring may be desirable but needs to be performed in a manner that avoids significant patient stress or significant respiratory compromise and hypoventilation from sedation.

The intraoperative care for patients with both significant carotid and coronary disease requires balancing the sometimes conflicting hemodynamic needs of these 2 disease processes. Optimal blood pressure management, for instance, requires careful monitoring of both organ systems (see monitoring section later). During isolated open carotid surgery, one technique to maintain cerebral perfusion pressure in the setting of carotid clamping is to use induced hypertension.[51] Assuming an intact circle of Willis circulation, augmenting mean artery pressure greater than baseline during carotid cross-clamping may provide collateral circulation to cerebral tissue at risk for ischemia. In combined carotid-coronary procedures, particularly if carotid revascularization is performed before the initiation of CPB, the use of this technique requires careful attention in order to avoid potential myocardial ischemia (eg, electrocardiogram [EKG] ST segment changes or wall motion changes on transesophageal echocardiography [TEE]). If empiric, induced hypertensive blood pressure goals (eg, 10%–20% greater than baseline during carotid cross-clamping) are not tolerated, blood pressure goals should be adjusted using guidance from cerebral monitoring techniques (eg, raw electroencephalogram [EEG]/somatosensory evoked potential [SSEP], processed EEG, cerebral oximetry) or carotid shunt placement (if not already used) may be necessary to help maintain cerebral perfusion while avoiding myocardial ischemic consequences.

In addition to optimizing cerebral blood flow, hemodynamics should be managed to optimize coronary blood flow and minimize myocardial oxygen demand. Intravenous nitroglycerine infusion can promote coronary vasodilation, decrease left ventricular preload and wall tension, and, thus, help balance myocardial oxygen supply and demand. Heart rate should be managed to avoid tachycardia, while at the same time avoiding significant bradycardia that might negatively impact cardiac output (ie, cardiac output = heart rate × stroke volume). Short-acting intravenous beta-blockade with metoprolol or an infusion of esmolol may be considered in patients with excessive heart rates and no contraindications to beta-blockade. If ischemia develops during carotid repair, early intervention is needed to avoid hemodynamic instability or ischemic arrhythmias. In cases of refractory ischemia or hemodynamic instability, early initiation of CPB or mechanical support with an intra-aortic balloon pump (IABP) should be considered. In certain high-risk individuals, IABP may be placed prophylactically at the beginning of the case.

EKG monitoring

A 5-lead EKG is standard and allows dysrhythmia identification and continuous ST-segment monitoring for detection of myocardial ischemia intraoperatively and postoperatively.

Hemodynamic monitoring

Similar to monitoring in the setting of isolated CABG, patients undergoing combined coronary revascularization generally warrant invasive monitoring of systemic arterial pressures and central filling pressures. Additionally, placement of a pulmonary artery catheter can provide measurements of cardiac filling and cardiac output. No consensus exists as to the benefit of routine utilization of pulmonary artery catheterization in CABG.[22] Routine placement of pulmonary artery catheter (PAC) varies depending on practice setting. The ACCF/AHA's guidelines do recommend the placement of a PAC in patients with cardiogenic shock, preferably before anesthesia induction (class I, evidence C) and perioperatively in hemodynamically unstable patients (class IIA, evidence B). In the setting of combined carotid and coronary revascularization procedures, the location of central catheters needs to be considered to avoid interference with the surgical procedure or recent carotid interventions (eg, cannulation of subclavian or contralateral internal jugular vein may be necessary).

TEE

Intraoperative TEE has become a standard monitoring method in cardiac surgery. The relative safety and incredible versatility of this technology makes it a highly valuable intraoperative monitoring and diagnostic tool.[52,53] In the setting of combined carotid and coronary intervention, TEE is particularly useful for monitoring for myocardial ischemia by providing real-time imaging of wall motion changes. TEE monitoring provides rapid information on global and regional myocardial function during the carotid portion of the procedure but also allows for the assessment of coronary graft function immediately after separation from CPB. Additionally, TEE can provide valuable imaging of the ascending and descending aorta and arch to evaluate for pathologic conditions, including dissection, aneurysm, and atherosclerotic disease.

Epiaortic scanning of the ascending aorta

Epiaortic scanning involves the direct scanning of the ascending aorta and arch to evaluate for the presence, location, and severity of atherosclerotic disease. Epiaortic scanning allows for visualization of both calcified and noncalcified plaques and has been shown to be at least two times more sensitive for aortic atherosclerotic disease than surgical examination and palpation.[54] Epiaortic ultrasound-guided aortic manipulation seems to be associated with decreased perioperative stroke[54–58] and is now recommended in the ACCF/AHA's 2011 guidelines for CABG procedures (class IIa, evidence B). Scanning is performed with a handheld probe in the surgical field, placed directly onto the ascending aorta, usually with a saline standoff (eg, saline-filled glove or probe sheath or saline flooding of the pericardium). The saline standoff improves the acoustic interface and allows for better visualization of the near-field aortic wall. A disadvantage of scanning is that it can only be performed intraoperatively, after chest opening, and, thus, requires a small surgical delay and a theoretic risk of infection. Given the apparent value of ascending aortic scanning to help decrease atherosclerotic emboli, efforts are being made to explore alternative imaging techniques. One device currently being studied is the A-View catheter (Cordatec Inc, Zoersel, Belgium), a saline-filled catheter that is placed in the left mainstem bronchus to eliminate echo interference associated with this structure and improve TEE imaging of the ascending aorta.[59,60]

Cerebral monitoring

Given the increased risk of adverse neurologic events associated with concomitant carotid and coronary disease, cerebral monitoring is an important consideration. In the setting of isolated CEA, cerebral monitoring techniques are widely used. During

CEA, cerebral monitoring can identify cerebral ischemia after carotid cross-clamping to help determine the need for carotid shunt placement. Although some practitioners opt for routine shunt placement to avoid the need for monitoring, others argue that shunting is associated with the risk of morbidity (eg, vascular dissection, embolization of air or plaque) and suggest selective shunting is preferred. Regardless of technique, many argue that cerebral monitoring should be routine in all carotid revascularization procedures in order to identify the cerebral condition and new neurologic events that require urgent intervention (eg, surgical management changes caused by the detection of embolic phenomena or shunt malfunction).[61]

Several cerebral monitoring modalities exist and include EEG monitoring, SSEP monitoring, and transcranial Doppler (TCD) as well as, more recently, monitoring of cortical oxygenation with near-infrared spectroscopy (NIRS) and utilization of processed EEG systems. The goal of cerebral monitoring is to identify hypoperfusion, embolic phenomena, and hyperperfusion states, all of which can be associated with perioperative stroke. Because no single monitoring technique is comprehensive, optimal monitoring requires a combination of modalities.

Electrophysiologic monitoring

The most common electrophysiologic monitoring modalities used in the setting of carotid revascularization are EEG and SSEP.

EEG is a summative measurement of spontaneous electrical activity of the cerebral cortex as detected by surface scalp electrodes.[62,63] Brain function is assessed by monitoring changes in the wave patterns generated by cortical electrical activity. Changes in electrical patterns are assessed and compared with the baseline as well as with the contralateral cerebral hemisphere. Significant changes in the EEG recording, such as more than a 50% decrease in amplitude of 8 to 15 Hz activity, are associated with cerebral ischemia and increased risk of stroke.[64] EEG is currently the most studied, best-established cerebral monitoring technique in the setting of carotid surgery.

Given the sensitivity of EEG to anesthetic agents, EEG monitoring is generally supplemented with concurrent SSEP monitoring, which has a more durable signal in the setting of anesthesia. SSEPs measure cortical responses to peripheral stimuli to identify compromises to cortical blood flow. Ischemia results in more than a 50% reduction in amplitude of the cortical response. For example, a stimulus to the median nerve would show a 50% reduction in amplitude from the baseline in the setting of cerebral hypoperfusion in the middle cerebral artery territory. However, because SSEPs cover only limited regions of the cortex, this monitoring method is not generally used in isolation. Although SSEP with concurrent EEG monitoring is frequently used in carotid revascularization, some question the reliability of SSEP to detect ischemia, arguing that studies have demonstrated large variability in sensitivity and specificity for SSEPs for predicting the need for shunt placement.[61,65,66]

TCD

TCD has also been widely used to monitor for cerebral ischemia. This technique uses continuous, noninvasive Doppler assessment of flow velocities in the large intracranial arteries. Decreases in blood flow are associated with lower cerebral perfusion. Additionally, TCD can detect embolic phenomena (ie, microembolic signals). This method is reliable and repeatable; however, it depends highly on operator/interpreter skill and is technically not feasible in approximately 10% to 15% patients because of the inability to achieve quality temporal bone ultrasound monitoring frames. TCD is unique in that it can also detect significant increases in cerebral blood flow associated with excessive cerebral perfusion that can occur after carotid revascularization. Early detection of significant hyperperfusion can allow for early intervention and treatment of hyperperfusion syndrome and may help reduce the risk of postoperative hemorrhagic stroke associated with this condition.[67] Additionally, TCD can be useful in identifying intracranial stenosis, which may also play a role in perioperative stroke in the setting of combined carotid coronary surgery.

Cerebral oximetry

NIRS is a noninvasive, nonpulsatile, continuous measure of regional cerebral oxygenation (rSO_2).[68] Sensors on the forehead sample oxygen saturation of the frontal cerebral cortex to assess perfusion.[69] NIRS-derived rSO_2 has been correlated with jugular venous bulb saturation,[70] and low rSO_2 (<45% absolute or >25% declines) are associated with poor neurologic outcomes after CABG surgery. Additionally, NIRS monitoring has been used to identify cannula malposition during cardiopulmonary bypass.[71]

Although there has been interest in NIRS monitoring to identify significant cerebral ischemia in the setting of carotid surgery, there is still considerable debate about the utility and reliability of this monitor for cerebral ischemia.[72] Available studies have shown some correlation but have demonstrated a low positive predictive value[73–75]; currently, no clear, reliable thresholds have been identified.[72] Furthermore, NIRS monitoring, as generally used, is limited to only the anterior portion of the frontal lobe, potentially missing perfusion compromises in other cerebral territories.[61] Additionally, some investigators question whether the saturations reflected by NIRS actually reflects cerebral tissue at all or whether the signal is too contaminated by superficial, extracranial tissue signals to be a reliable monitor of cerebral oxygenation.[73] Despite the advantages this mode of monitoring offers, such as being relatively easy to use, not being user dependent, and having good temporal resolution, there are still important unresolved questions about how to apply this technology.

Processed EEG

In contrast to raw EEG, bispectral index (BIS), a processed EEG primarily used to predict anesthetic depth, has been suggested as a monitor for unilateral decreases in cerebral blood flow. BIS uses various algorithms to translate the EEG signature into an indexed score (0–100).[63,76] Although the clinical utility of these numeric values is debated,[73,75] the EEG data do provide an opportunity to compare cortical activity between the hemispheres. Nevertheless, studies of BIS in the setting of CEA have had low predictive value for cerebral ischemia; it is generally not recommended as a primary monitoring modality.[61]

Intensive Care Unit Considerations

Postoperative considerations for patients undergoing combined carotid revascularization and CABG are generally similar to post-CABG patients; therefore, all aspects of intensive care unit (ICU) management are not reviewed here. This patient population, however, does present a few unique management issues that should be considered.

Postoperative stroke and MI

Given the generally higher surgical risk profile associated with the patient population that is likely to undergo combined carotid/CABG,[77] these patients warrant careful monitoring for signs of postoperative stroke or MI.

Cerebral hyperemia/cerebral hyperperfusion syndrome

Carotid revascularization can be complicated by postprocedure cerebral hyperperfusion/hyperemia. Cerebral hyperperfusion syndrome (CHS), a triad of ipsilateral headache, transient focal neurologic deficit, and seizure without compromised cerebral blood flow, is associated with impaired autoregulation and hemorrhagic stroke.[78] Approximately 1% to 3% of CEA is complicated by CHS[61]; cerebral hemorrhage in this setting is associated with a 40% mortality risk.[61] With hyperperfusion, cerebral blood flow is observed to exceed 100% of normal values and can be diagnosed with computed tomography (CT)/single-photon emission CT imaging.[79] In the context of combined carotid/CABG procedures, the need to maintain adequate blood pressures to ensure coronary graft perfusion must be balanced against hyperperfusion of the carotid/cerebral vascular bed and the associated risk of intracranial hemorrhage. Additionally, neurologic monitoring may be complicated by slow emergence after cardiac procedures. When possible, anesthetic techniques that favor rapid emergence and extubation are preferable to allow for early identification of adverse cerebral events.

Bleeding

According to the society of thoracic surgeons database, 2.4% of isolated CABG patients require reoperation for bleeding after initial surgery.[80] In the setting of combined CEA/CABG, the usual complications of postoperative hemorrhage (eg, tamponade, hypovolemia, coagulopathy) must be considered in addition to the risk of cervical hematoma and related airway compromise. Although early emergence and extubation in this population is desirable to allow for monitoring of neurologic status, careful attention to the cervical wound and airway patency is essential.

If carotid stenting is used for carotid revascularization, postoperative hematologic management must balance the need for surgical hemostasis with the need for antiplatelet therapy to prevent stent thrombosis. Typically, anticoagulation with thienopyridine is initiated 6 or more hours after surgery in the absence of acute bleeding.[81–83] However, given the increased risk of bleeding associated with these agents in the CAS/CABG population, vigilance is necessary to recognize early signs of postoperative hemorrhage in these patients.

SUMMARY

As the general population ages, the prevalence of severe carotid atherosclerotic disease is increasing in the patient population presenting for coronary artery bypass. Estimates suggest that significant carotid stenosis (>70%) is now present in close to 10% of the CABG population. As a result, the need to manage patients with significant concurrent stenosis of the carotid and coronary arteries is likely to become more common in the future. Although many questions still remain about the optimal surgical approach to this high-risk patient population, it is clear that these patients, when they do present in the surgical amphitheatre, present important clinical anesthetic challenges.

REFERENCES

1. Roffi M, Ribichini F, Castriota F, et al. Management of combined severe carotid and coronary artery disease. Curr Cardiol Rep 2012;14(2):125–34.
2. Naylor AR, Cuffe RL, Rothwell PM, et al. A systematic review of outcomes following staged and synchronous carotid endarterectomy and coronary artery bypass. Eur J Vasc Endovasc Surg 2003;25(5):380–9.
3. Prasad SM, Li S, Rankin JS, et al. Current outcomes of simultaneous carotid endarterectomy and coronary artery bypass graft surgery in North America. World J Surg 2010;34(10):2292–8.

4. Stamou SC, Hill PC, Dangas G, et al. Stroke after coronary artery bypass: incidence, predictors, and clinical outcome. Stroke 2001;32(7):1508–13.
5. Merie C, Kober L, Olsen PS, et al. Risk of stroke after coronary artery bypass grafting: effect of age and comorbidities. Stroke 2012;43(1):38–43.
6. Naylor AR, Mehta Z, Rothwell PM, et al. Carotid artery disease and stroke during coronary artery bypass: a critical review of the literature. Eur J Vasc Endovasc Surg 2002;23(4):283–94.
7. Tarakji KG, Sabik JF, Bhudia SK, et al. Temporal onset, risk factors, and outcomes associated with stroke after coronary artery bypass grafting. JAMA 2011;305(4):381–90.
8. Naylor AR. Asymptomatic carotid artery stenosis: state of the art management. J Cardiovasc Surg (Torino) 2013;54(1 Suppl 1):1–7.
9. Likosky DS, Marrin CA, Caplan LR, et al. Determination of etiologic mechanisms of strokes secondary to coronary artery bypass graft surgery. Stroke 2003; 34(12):2830–4.
10. Macdonald S. Brain injury secondary to carotid intervention. J Endovasc Ther 2007;14(2):219–31.
11. Belden JR, Caplan LR, Pessin MS, et al. Mechanisms and clinical features of posterior border-zone infarcts. Neurology 1999;53(6):1312–8.
12. Roach GW, Kanchuger M, Mangano CM, et al. Adverse cerebral outcomes after coronary bypass surgery. N Engl J Med 1996;335(25):1857–64.
13. D'Agostino RS, Svensson LG, Neumann DJ, et al. Screening carotid ultrasonography and risk factors for stroke in coronary artery surgery patients. Ann Thorac Surg 1996;62(6):1714–23.
14. Tuman KJ, McCarthy RJ, Najafi H, et al. Differential effects of advanced age on neurologic and cardiac risks of coronary artery operations. J Thorac Cardiovasc Surg 1992;104(6):1510–7.
15. Fairhead JF, Mehta Z, Rothwell PM. Population-based study of delays in carotid imaging and surgery and the risk of recurrent stroke. Neurology 2005;65(3): 371–5.
16. Naylor AR. Synchronous cardiac and carotid revascularisation: the devil is in the detail. Eur J Vasc Endovasc Surg 2010;40(3):303–8.
17. Venkatachalam S, Shishehbor MH. Management of carotid disease in patients undergoing coronary artery bypass surgery: is it time to change our approach? Curr Opin Cardiol 2011;26(6):480–7.
18. Venkatachalam S, Gray BH, Mukherjee D, et al. Contemporary management of concomitant carotid and coronary artery disease. Heart 2011;97(3):175–80.
19. Durand DJ, Perler BA, Roseborough GS, et al. Mandatory versus selective preoperative carotid screening: a retrospective analysis. Ann Thorac Surg 2004; 78(1):159–66 [discussion: 159–66].
20. Sheiman RG, Janne d'Othee B. Screening carotid sonography before elective coronary artery bypass graft surgery: who needs it. AJR Am J Roentgenol 2007;188(5):W475–9.
21. Brott TG, Halperin JL, Abbara S, et al. 2011 ASA/ACCF/AHA/AANN/AANS/ACR/ ASNR/CNS/SAIP/SCAI/SIR/SNIS/SVM/SVS guideline on the management of patients with extracranial carotid and vertebral artery disease. A report of the American College of Cardiology Foundation/American Heart Association task force on practice guidelines, and the American Stroke Association, American Association of Neuroscience Nurses, American Association of Neurological Surgeons, American College of Radiology, American Society of Neuroradiology, Congress of Neurological Surgeons, Society of Atherosclerosis Imaging and

Prevention, Society for Cardiovascular Angiography and Interventions, Society of Interventional Radiology, Society of NeuroInterventional Surgery, Society for Vascular Medicine, and Society for Vascular Surgery. Circulation 2011;124(4):e54–130.

22. Hillis LD, Smith PK, Anderson JL, et al. Special articles: 2011 ACCF/AHA guideline for coronary artery bypass graft surgery: executive summary: a report of the American College of Cardiology Foundation/American Heart Association task force on practice guidelines. Anesth Analg 2012;114(1):11–45.
23. Li Y, Walicki D, Mathiesen C, et al. Strokes after cardiac surgery and relationship to carotid stenosis. Arch Neurol 2009;66(9):1091–6.
24. Lee EJ, Choi KH, Ryu JS, et al. Stroke risk after coronary artery bypass graft surgery and extent of cerebral artery atherosclerosis. J Am Coll Cardiol 2011;57(18):1811–8.
25. Naylor AR, Bown MJ. Stroke after cardiac surgery and its association with asymptomatic carotid disease: an updated systematic review and meta-analysis. Eur J Vasc Endovasc Surg 2011;41(5):607–24.
26. Venkatachalam S, Gray BH, Shishehbor MH. Open and endovascular management of concomitant severe carotid and coronary artery disease: tabular review of the literature. Ann Vasc Surg 2012;26(1):125–40.
27. Gopaldas RR, Chu D, Dao TK, et al. Staged versus synchronous carotid endarterectomy and coronary artery bypass grafting: analysis of 10-year nationwide outcomes. Ann Thorac Surg 2011;91(5):1323–9 [discussion: 1329].
28. Naylor AR. Time to rethink management strategies in asymptomatic carotid artery disease. Nat Rev Cardiol 2011;9(2):116–24.
29. Jones DW, Stone DH, Conrad MF, et al. Regional use of combined carotid endarterectomy/coronary artery bypass graft and the effect of patient risk. J Vasc Surg 2012;56(3):668–76.
30. Brooks WH, Jones MR, Gisler P, et al. Carotid angioplasty with stenting versus endarterectomy: 10-year randomized trial in a community hospital. JACC Cardiovasc Interv 2014;7(2):163–8.
31. Brott TG, Hobson RW, Howard G, et al. Stenting versus endarterectomy for treatment of carotid-artery stenosis. N Engl J Med 2010;363(1):11–23.
32. Usman AA, Tang GL, Eskandari MK. Meta-analysis of procedural stroke and death among octogenarians: carotid stenting versus carotid endarterectomy. J Am Coll Surg 2009;208(6):1124–31.
33. Gurm HS, Yadav JS, Fayad P, et al. Long-term results of carotid stenting versus endarterectomy in high-risk patients. N Engl J Med 2008;358(15):1572–9.
34. Guzman LA, Costa MA, Angiolillo DJ, et al. A systematic review of outcomes in patients with staged carotid artery stenting and coronary artery bypass graft surgery. Stroke 2008;39(2):361–5.
35. Nurozler F, Kutlu T, Kucuk G, et al. Impact of clopidogrel on postoperative blood loss after non-elective coronary bypass surgery. Interact Cardiovasc Thorac Surg 2005;4(6):546–9.
36. Ricotta JJ, Aburahma A, Ascher E, et al. Updated Society for Vascular Surgery guidelines for management of extracranial carotid disease. J Vasc Surg 2011;54(3):e1–31.
37. Furie KL, Kasner SE, Adams RJ, et al. Guidelines for the prevention of stroke in patients with stroke or transient ischemic attack: a guideline for healthcare professionals from the American Heart Association/American Stroke Association. Stroke 2011;42(1):227–76.

38. Chalmers J, Todd A, Chapman N, et al. International Society of Hypertension (ISH): statement on blood pressure lowering and stroke prevention. J Hypertens 2003;21(4):651–63.
39. POISE Study Group, Devereaux PJ, Yang H, et al. Effects of extended-release metoprolol succinate in patients undergoing non-cardiac surgery (POISE trial): a randomised controlled trial. Lancet 2008;371(9627):1839–47.
40. McGirt MJ, Perler BA, Brooke BS, et al. 3-hydroxy-3-methylglutaryl coenzyme A reductase inhibitors reduce the risk of perioperative stroke and mortality after carotid endarterectomy. J Vasc Surg 2005;42(5):829–36 [discussion: 836–7].
41. Amarenco P, Labreuche J. Lipid management in the prevention of stroke: review and updated meta-analysis of statins for stroke prevention. Lancet Neurol 2009; 8(5):453–63.
42. Baigent C, Keech A, Kearney PM, et al. Efficacy and safety of cholesterol-lowering treatment: prospective meta-analysis of data from 90,056 participants in 14 randomised trials of statins. Lancet 2005;366(9493):1267–78.
43. Liakopoulos OJ, Choi YH, Haldenwang PL, et al. Impact of preoperative statin therapy on adverse postoperative outcomes in patients undergoing cardiac surgery: a meta-analysis of over 30,000 patients. Eur Heart J 2008;29(12):1548–59.
44. Lau WC, Froehlich JB, Jewell ES, et al. Impact of adding aspirin to beta-blocker and statin in high-risk patients undergoing major vascular surgery. Ann Vasc Surg 2013;27(4):537–45.
45. Mangano DT, Multicenter Study of Perioperative Ischemia Research Group. Aspirin and mortality from coronary bypass surgery. N Engl J Med 2002; 347(17):1309–17.
46. Bybee KA, Powell BD, Valeti U, et al. Preoperative aspirin therapy is associated with improved postoperative outcomes in patients undergoing coronary artery bypass grafting. Circulation 2005;112(Suppl 9):I286–92.
47. Wright RS, Anderson JL, Adams CD, et al. 2011 ACCF/AHA focused update of the guidelines for the management of patients with unstable angina/non-ST-elevation myocardial infarction (updating the 2007 guideline): a report of the American College of Cardiology Foundation/American Heart Association Task Force on practice guidelines developed in collaboration with the American College of Emergency Physicians, Society for Cardiovascular Angiography and Interventions, and Society of Thoracic Surgeons. J Am Coll Cardiol 2011;57(19): 1920–59.
48. Anderson JL, Adams CD, Antman EM, et al. 2012 ACCF/AHA focused update incorporated into the ACCF/AHA 2007 guidelines for the management of patients with unstable angina/non-ST-elevation myocardial infarction: a report of the American College of Cardiology Foundation/American Heart Association task force on practice guidelines. J Am Coll Cardiol 2013;61(23):e179–347.
49. Slogoff S, Keats AS, Dear WE, et al. Steal-prone coronary anatomy and myocardial ischemia associated with four primary anesthetic agents in humans. Anesth Analg 1991;72(1):22–7.
50. Tuman KJ, McCarthy RJ, Spiess BD, et al. Does choice of anesthetic agent significantly affect outcome after coronary artery surgery? Anesthesiology 1989;70(2):189–98.
51. LeSar CJ, Sprouse LR, Harris WB. Permissive hypertension during awake eversion carotid endarterectomy: a physiologic approach for cerebral protection. J Am Coll Surg 2014;218(4):760–6.
52. Hilberath JN, Oakes DA, Shernan SK, et al. Safety of transesophageal echocardiography. J Am Soc Echocardiogr 2010;23(11):1115–27 [quiz: 1220–1].

53. Reeves ST, Finley AC, Skubas NJ, et al. Basic perioperative transesophageal echocardiography examination: a consensus statement of the American Society of Echocardiography and the Society of Cardiovascular Anesthesiologists. J Am Soc Echocardiogr 2013;26(5):443–56.
54. Marshall WG Jr, Barzilai B, Kouchoukos NT, et al. Intraoperative ultrasonic imaging of the ascending aorta. Ann Thorac Surg 1989;48(3):339–44.
55. Glas KE, Swaminathan M, Reeves ST, et al. Guidelines for the performance of a comprehensive intraoperative epiaortic ultrasonographic examination: recommendations of the American Society of Echocardiography and the Society of Cardiovascular Anesthesiologists; endorsed by the Society of Thoracic Surgeons. Anesth Analg 2008;106(5):1376–84.
56. Nakamura M, Okamoto F, Nakanishi K, et al. Does intensive management of cerebral hemodynamics and atheromatous aorta reduce stroke after coronary artery surgery? Ann Thorac Surg 2008;85(2):513–9.
57. Yamaguchi A, Adachi H, Tanaka M, et al. Efficacy of intraoperative epiaortic ultrasound scanning for preventing stroke after coronary artery bypass surgery. Ann Thorac Cardiovasc Surg 2009;15(2):98–104.
58. Rosenberger P, Shernan SK, Loffler M, et al. The influence of epiaortic ultrasonography on intraoperative surgical management in 6051 cardiac surgical patients. Ann Thorac Surg 2008;85(2):548–53.
59. van Zaane B, Nierich AP, Buhre WF, et al. Resolving the blind spot of transoesophageal echocardiography: a new diagnostic device for visualizing the ascending aorta in cardiac surgery. Br J Anaesth 2007;98(4):434–41.
60. Grocott HP, Tran T. Aortic atheroma and adverse cerebral outcome: risk, diagnosis, and management options. Semin Cardiothorac Vasc Anesth 2010;14(2):86–94.
61. Pennekamp CW, Bots ML, Kappelle LJ, et al. The value of near-infrared spectroscopy measured cerebral oximetry during carotid endarterectomy in perioperative stroke prevention. A review. Eur J Vasc Endovasc Surg 2009;38(5):539–45.
62. Rampil IJ. A primer for EEG signal processing in anesthesia. Anesthesiology 1998;89(4):980–1002.
63. Al-Kadi MI, Reaz MB, Ali MA. Evolution of electroencephalogram signal analysis techniques during anesthesia. Sensors (Basel) 2013;13(5):6605–35.
64. Isley MR, Edmonds HL Jr, Stecker M, American Society of Neurophysiological Monitoring. Guidelines for intraoperative neuromonitoring using raw (analog or digital waveforms) and quantitative electroencephalography: a position statement by the American Society of Neurophysiological Monitoring. J Clin Monit Comput 2009;23(6):369–90.
65. Fielmuth S, Uhlig T. The role of somatosensory evoked potentials in detecting cerebral ischaemia during carotid endarterectomy. Eur J Anaesthesiol 2008; 25(8):648–56.
66. Liu H, Di Giorgio AM, Williams ES, et al. Protocol for electrophysiological monitoring of carotid endarterectomies. J Biomed Res 2010;24(6):460–6.
67. Rodriguez RA, Rubens FD, Wozny D, et al. Cerebral emboli detected by transcranial Doppler during cardiopulmonary bypass are not correlated with postoperative cognitive deficits. Stroke 2010;41(10):2229–35.
68. Scheeren TW, Schober P, Schwarte LA. Monitoring tissue oxygenation by near infrared spectroscopy (NIRS): background and current applications. J Clin Monit Comput 2012;26(4):279–87.
69. Murkin JM, Adams SJ, Novick RJ, et al. Monitoring brain oxygen saturation during coronary bypass surgery: a randomized, prospective study. Anesth Analg 2007;104(1):51–8.

70. Kim MB, Ward DS, Cartwright CR, et al. Estimation of jugular venous O2 saturation from cerebral oximetry or arterial O2 saturation during isocapnic hypoxia. J Clin Monit Comput 2000;16(3):191–9.
71. Zheng F, Sheinberg R, Yee MS, et al. Cerebral near-infrared spectroscopy monitoring and neurologic outcomes in adult cardiac surgery patients: a systematic review. Anesth Analg 2013;116(3):663–76.
72. Ghosh A, Elwell C, Smith M. Review article: cerebral near-infrared spectroscopy in adults: a work in progress. Anesth Analg 2012;115(6):1373–83.
73. Miyazawa T, Horiuchi M, Komine H, et al. Skin blood flow influences cerebral oxygenation measured by near-infrared spectroscopy during dynamic exercise. Eur J Appl Physiol 2013;113(11):2841–8.
74. Mauermann WJ, Crepeau AZ, Pulido JN, et al. Comparison of electroencephalography and cerebral oximetry to determine the need for in-line arterial shunting in patients undergoing carotid endarterectomy. J Cardiothorac Vasc Anesth 2013;27(6):1253–9.
75. Samra SK, Dy EA, Welch K, et al. Evaluation of a cerebral oximeter as a monitor of cerebral ischemia during carotid endarterectomy. Anesthesiology 2000;93(4): 964–70.
76. Sury M. Brain monitoring in children. Anesthesiol Clin 2014;32(1):115–32.
77. Timaran CH, Rosero EB, Smith ST, et al. Trends and outcomes of concurrent carotid revascularization and coronary bypass. J Vasc Surg 2008;48(2): 355–60 [discussion: 360–1].
78. Moulakakis KG, Mylonas SN, Sfyroeras GS, et al. Hyperperfusion syndrome after carotid revascularization. J Vasc Surg 2009;49(4):1060–8.
79. Kaku Y, Yoshimura S, Kokuzawa J. Factors predictive of cerebral hyperperfusion after carotid angioplasty and stent placement. AJNR Am J Neuroradiol 2004; 25(8):1403–8.
80. Mehta RH, Sheng S, O'Brien SM, et al. Reoperation for bleeding in patients undergoing coronary artery bypass surgery: incidence, risk factors, time trends, and outcomes. Circ Cardiovasc Qual Outcomes 2009;2(6):583–90.
81. Van der Heyden J, Suttorp MJ, Bal ET, et al. Staged carotid angioplasty and stenting followed by cardiac surgery in patients with severe asymptomatic carotid artery stenosis: early and long-term results. Circulation 2007;116(18): 2036–42.
82. Mendiz OA, Fava CM, Lev GA, et al. Hybrid strategy for unstable patients with severe carotid and cardiac disease requiring surgery. Cardiol J 2014. [Epub ahead of print].
83. Abbasi K, Fadaei Araghi M, Zafarghandi M, et al. Concomitant carotid endarterectomy and coronary artery bypass grafting versus staged carotid stenting followed by coronary artery bypass grafting. J Cardiovasc Surg (Torino) 2008; 49(2):285–8.

Considerations for Patients Undergoing Endovascular Abdominal Aortic Aneurysm Repair

Brant W. Ullery, MD, Jason T. Lee, MD*

KEYWORDS

• Endovascular aneurysm repair • Fenestrated stent-grafts • Thoracic stent-grafts

KEY POINTS

- Endovascular aneurysm repair has replaced open surgery for most elective and urgent repair of anatomically suitable aortic aneurysms.
- Risk factors for anesthetic complications after endovascular aneurysm repair are related to cardiac comorbidities, chronic obstructive pulmonary disease, and renal function.
- Perioperative management strategies must include careful attention to fluid status, renal protection, spinal cord perfusion, and hemodynamic stability during procedures.

INTRODUCTION

Since the introduction of endovascular aneurysm repair (EVAR) by Parodi and colleagues in 1991[1] and the subsequent approval of early endovascular devices by the US Food and Drug Administration in 1999, EVAR has gained widespread acceptance as the procedure of choice for patients with infrarenal abdominal aortic aneurysms (AAAs) and suitable aortic anatomy. The shift toward a less-invasive approach to the surgical management of AAAs reflects a national trend in both training and practice patterns, with one recent report citing EVAR to comprise more than two-thirds of all AAA repairs.[2,3] Such trends are likely to continue well into the foreseeable future as subsequent generations of stent-grafts expand the applicability of EVAR to patients with more challenging anatomy and therefore more physiologic compromise. EVAR has been demonstrated to be safer and as durable a therapeutic alternative to conventional open AAA repair in prospective national and international trials.[4–7] Indeed, the development and increasing utilization of more advanced endovascular techniques

Division of Vascular Surgery, Stanford University Medical Center, 300 Pasteur Drive, H3600, Stanford, CA 94305, USA
* Corresponding author.
E-mail address: jtlee@stanford.edu

Anesthesiology Clin 32 (2014) 723–734
http://dx.doi.org/10.1016/j.anclin.2014.05.003 anesthesiology.theclinics.com

involving snorkel or periscope grafts and customized fenestrated and branched aortic stent grafts have radically expanded the scope of patients able to receive this form of treatment strategy, including select patients with complex juxtarenal, pararenal, and thoracoabdominal aortic aneurysms. Understanding these alternatives and how the physiologic stressors can be potentially different in EVAR versus open repair become an important consideration for anesthesia providers.

INDICATIONS

Clinical management of AAAs is guided by the risk of aneurysm rupture, perceived perioperative morality risk, life expectancy, and patient preference. The single most important parameter associated with rupture is maximal cross-sectional aneurysm diameter. Risk of rupture is estimated at 1% to 3% per year for aneurysms of 4 to 5 cm, 6% to 11% per year for aneurysms of 5 to 7 cm, and 20% per year for aneurysms larger than 7 cm. In addition to aneurysm size, rupture risk also has been shown to be increased among women, as well as in patients with chronic obstructive pulmonary disease, tobacco use, and hypertension.[8] EVAR is generally recommended once aneurysm size reaches a specific threshold, typically 4.5 to 5.0 cm in women and 5.0 to 5.5 cm in men. Symptomatic (eg, abdominal or back pain) aneurysms of any size or those exhibiting rapid growth of more than 0.5 cm within a period of 6 months represent additional indications for EVAR because of an associated increase in risk of rupture.

Perioperative morality risk also must be weighed against the potential rupture risk. Independent risk factors for perioperative mortality among patients undergoing AAA repair include congestive heart failure, increased age, female gender, renal insufficiency, and myocardial ischemia.[9] Patients should generally have an estimated life expectancy of more than 2 years to benefit from the survival advantage of undergoing EVAR. A recent study demonstrated that 84% of patients with AAAs would prefer endovascular repair in lieu of conventional open surgery, even despite concerns pertaining to long-term outcome.[10]

In addition to clinical indications, anatomic suitability of AAAs for endovascular repair is of critical importance to optimize therapeutic efficacy via successful aneurysm exclusion. Aneurysm morphology and anatomic measurements are most commonly assessed using 3-dimensional reconstructions from computed tomographic angiography. Features of aneurysms commonly assessed include, most importantly, the length, diameter, and angulation of the proximal neck, as well as variables related to the tortuosity, degree of intraluminal thrombus, size of access vessels, and length and diameter of the distal landing zone. Each stent graft device is accompanied by specific instructions for use from the manufacturer, which details anatomic requirements needed to safely implant the stent graft and successfully exclude the aneurysm.

To ensure adequate proximal fixation, proximal aneurysm necks generally should be smaller than 30 mm in diameter, have 4 to 15 mm of neck length (dependent on device chosen to use), and be relatively free from significant calcification or thrombus. Proximal neck angulation, defined as the angle between the suprarenal aorta and the first portion of the aneurysm neck, should ideally be less than 45° to 60°, although newer-generation devices are challenging even this requirement. Last, iliofemoral access vessels, which become a concern for potential blood loss and anesthetic concerns, should have a minimum diameter of 6 to 8 mm to accommodate the sheaths required (often up to 24F) to advance and deploy the aortic stent-grafts. With increasing surgeon experience, however, EVAR has been performed in more challenging anatomies with excellent results even despite being outside the instructions for use.[11] As later-generation devices are being introduced and studied, the indications for EVAR are becoming broader. Newer endovascular technologies, including the recent development of fenestrated and branched endografts, are increasingly applied to the treatment of select patients with complex juxtarenal, suprarenal, and thoracoabdominal aneurysms.

CONTRAINDICATIONS

Disadvantageous anatomy of the proximal aneurysm neck serves as the most common contraindication for EVAR in more than 40% of cases.[12] Aneurysm neck diameters in excess of 30 mm are considered contraindications because the largest diameter of commercially available stent grafts is 36 mm and device oversizing of 10% to 20% is generally desired.[13] Inadequate aneurysm neck length (ie, generally less than 4 to 7 mm) prohibits adequate anchoring and fixation in a sufficient length of healthy proximal aorta, again dependent on the device. Proximal neck angulation of more than 60° and the presence of significant thrombus or calcification at the aneurysm neck also compromise successful proximal fixation of the aortic stent graft and increase the risk for stent migration, endoleak, or stent facture.

Small-caliber, heavily calcified iliofemoral vessels also serve as a contraindication for EVAR, given the associated risk for access-site related complications, including hemorrhage, pseudoaneurysm, dissection, or rupture. In the EUROSTAR registry, EVAR was unsuccessful in up to 13% of patients secondary to issues related to unfavorable access vessels.[14] There are several well-described techniques that may be used to assist in overcoming many of these access site–related limitations, including installation of a so-called buddy wire to straighten a tortuous iliac system or the surgical creation of aortic or iliac conduits.

PATIENT PREPARATION

EVAR is considered an intermediate-risk procedure according to the American College of Cardiology/American Heart Association guidelines.[15] Therefore, preoperative noninvasive testing is not required unless the patient is noted to have 2 or more clinical predictors of coronary ischemia. Severe coronary artery disease is present in 50% of patients in whom it is suspected and in 20% of patients without clinical indications of the disease. The use of dipyridamole (or Persantine) thallium cardiac scintillation scan or a dobutamine echocardiogram to select patients at risk for intraoperative ischemia guides which patients may benefit from preoperative catheter-based or surgical coronary revascularization. Particular patients at risk include older patients and those with a history of myocardial infarction, active angina pectoris, congestive heart failure, abnormal baseline electrocardiogram, and diabetes mellitus. Standard measures of perioperative cardiac risk include the use of Eagle risk criteria,[16] which been studied in EVAR populations and can provide preoperative prediction of cardiac-related complications based on certain criteria.

Other important risk factors for patients undergoing EVAR include chronic obstructive pulmonary disease and impaired renal function. As such, pulmonary function studies can serve as a rough prognostic guide and should be optimized before surgical intervention. Preoperative renal function is an important determinant of perioperative morbidity and may heavily influence the form and quantity of contrast agents in diagnostic tests or at the time of endovascular repair. Impaired renal function also may prompt some surgeons to perform EVAR under the guidance of intravascular ultrasound so as to dramatically decrease the exposure to nephrotoxic contrast agents.

TECHNIQUE BEST PRACTICES

Endovascular aneurysm repair differs from open surgical repair in that the prosthetic graft is introduced in the aneurysm through the femoral arteries and fixed in place to the nonaneurysmal infrarenal neck with self-expanding or balloon-expandable stents rather than sutures. A major abdominal incision is thus avoided and patient morbidity related to the procedure is theoretically reduced. The first endovascular aneurysm repair was performed in 1991 using a Dacron graft sutured onto balloon-expandable Palmaz stents.[1] The effectiveness of endovascular repair was demonstrated in the 1990s by using a variety of homemade devices. A number of commercially manufactured stent grafts have since been developed, with EVAR now representing the primary treatment modality for anatomically suitable patients. Randomized trials comparing open to endovascular techniques have been performed in Europe, with results demonstrating equivalent long-term survival and significantly reduced 30-day morbidity and mortality.[4–7]

Procedure

The technical details of endovascular repair vary with each specific device, but the general principles are similar. In most cases, a self-expanding stent graft is inserted into the aorta after open surgical or percutaneous exposure of both common femoral arteries. The femoral arteries are cannulated and guide wires are advanced into the aorta. Systemic heparinization is routinely performed after cannulation of the femoral arteries. Heparin is administered with a target activated clotting time (ACT) that is 2.0 to 2.5 times the baseline (approximately 250–300 seconds). Most stent grafts are made of 2 pieces: a main module including the body and one of the limbs with a gate for the separate contralateral limb. The appropriately sized primary module is inserted under fluoroscopic guidance and deployed immediately below the most caudal renal artery. The opening in the bifurcated module for the contralateral limb is deployed at this time, thereby unveiling the contralateral limb, which is cannulated from the corresponding ipsilateral femoral artery. Additional stent grafts, referred to as iliac limbs, are placed as needed in such a way that they overlap with the initial main body piece and land distally at the level of the distal common iliac arteries. After balloon molding the stent grafts to ensure adequate proximal, distal, and overlapping stent fixation, the aneurysm is fully excluded from systemic circulation (**Fig. 1**).

During no time of the procedure is a proximal cross-clamp necessary that would often require pharmacologic adjustment of blood pressure parameters. Balloon-molding of the main body endografts is often done over several seconds, causing only transient rise in systemic blood pressure. The overall physiologic insult to clamping and reperfusion seen so often in open aortic surgery is not present with EVAR.

Additional Advanced Endovascular Techniques

Fenestrated EVAR uses customized aortic prostheses with circular or elliptical holes, or fenestrations, in the side portion of the main body graft and U-shaped holes, referred to as scallops, in the proximal margin of the main body graft. The proximal main body stent graft component may accommodate a combination of up to 3 fenestrations or scallops, thereby maintaining visceral arterial patency and facilitating a more proximal sealing position compared with standard EVAR. Although the first report of a juxtarenal AAA treated with the use of a fenestrated stent graft was reported in 1999,[17] experience in the United States remains in its relative infancy, with few centers gaining access to either the clinical trial or investigation device exemption (IDE)-sponsored trials until the recent approval of the Zenith fenestrated endovascular

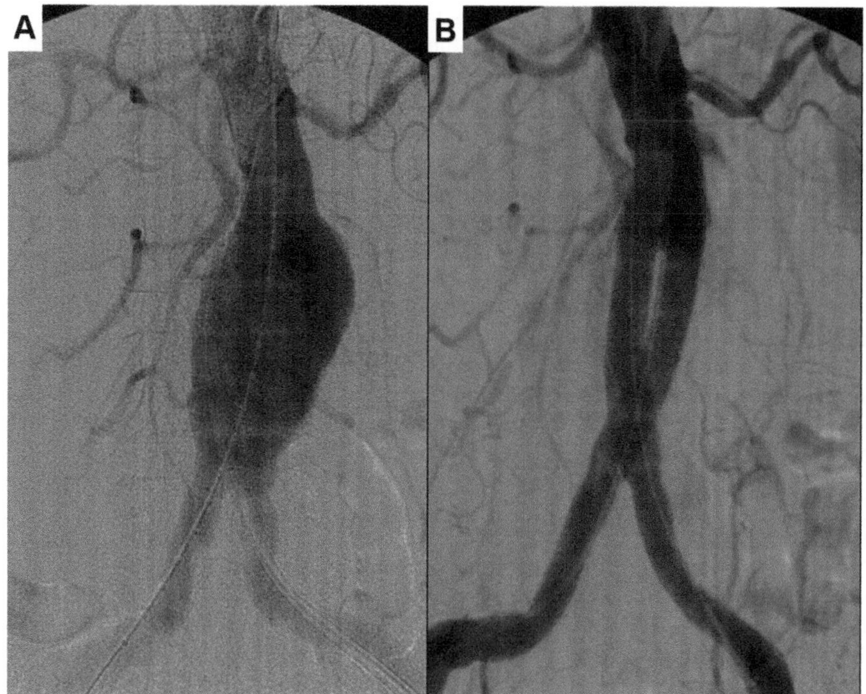

Fig. 1. Intraoperative angiogram of large 7-cm abdominal aortic aneurysm (*A*) before and (*B*) after successful placement of bifurcated stent-graft to provide exclusion.

(ZFEN) AAA device (Cook Medical, Bloomington, IN) by the Food and Drug Administration in April 2012. An increasing number of published series have demonstrated favorable early and mid-term results using this advanced endovascular technique.[18,19]

The fenestrated technique begins preoperatively with custom design of the scallop and fenestrations relative to clock positions and at chosen distances from the proximal edge of fabric. During the actual procedure, the proximal main body is introduced, with proper rotational orientation confirmed by the overlap of an anterior row of vertical and posterior row of horizontal markers to form a cross. Correct orientation also is confirmed with reference to the marginal radiopaque markers of the renal fenestrations and superior mesenteric artery scallop. Selective catheterization of the target visceral vessels is performed at this time and confirmed using a small-contrast medium injection. Sheaths are advanced into all target vessels, and prepositioning of stents within the sheaths, where applicable, is performed before endograft deployment. It is our practice to place covered stents within target vessels accommodated by small fenestrations. We do not routinely stent target vessels accommodated by either scallops or large fenestrations. The proximal main body graft is deployed at this time. Stents are flared approximately 5 mm within the aortic lumen to enhance fixation and minimize risk of endoleak. Completion angiography after assembly and deployment of all modular components is performed to document target vessel patency and presence of any endoleak.

The snorkel or chimney technique evolved because of the lack of readily available branched and fenestrated EVAR options. This technique uses only standard aortic stent grafts and therefore eliminates the manufacturing delays required for the customization of fenestrated stent grafts. In this technique, one or more stent-grafts are positioned in parallel to the main aortic stent graft so as to extend the proximal or distal sealing zone and maintain visceral arterial patency. These parallel grafts are positioned between the aortic wall and the main aortic stent graft in a cranial (snorkel) or caudal (periscope) direction. The target visceral vessels are catheterized from a femoral, brachial, or axillosubclavian approach, leading to additional considerations for patient positioning and the ability for the anesthesia team to use a left-sided arterial line, as well as left-sided central access. Discussion with the endovascular surgeon before the intervention is paramount in determining optimal anesthetic strategy for each individual patient. Stiff wires and covered stents are then placed into the proximal visceral vessels. Subsequently balloon dilation of the snorkel grafts is performed simultaneously with the main body stent-graft in a "kissing" fashion to ensure an optimal theoretic seal and minimization of "gutter" channels around each snorkel stent. After completion of the proximal portion of the procedure, angiography verifies no proximal type I endoleak, and the iliac limbs are then deployed in the standard fashion while maintaining wire access to the snorkel grafts.

Intraoperative Management

Radiation safety

Endovascular interventions have become a mainstay within the field of vascular surgery. The increased frequency and procedural complexity of these interventions, particularly with regard to EVAR, have forced vascular interventionalists and anesthesiologists alike to be faced with the ongoing risk of additional occupational radiation exposure. The cornerstones of radiation safety for the operating team revolve around time, distance, and shielding. Effort should be made by the anesthesia staff to maximize their distance from the radiation source and regularly wear effective radiation-protective shielding. The inverse square law states that radiation scatter will decrease by the square of the distance to source of radiation; therefore, doubling the distance from a point source of radiation will decrease the exposure rate to one-fourth the original exposure rate.

Renal protection

Given the required use of iodinated contrast medium during EVAR, preoperative renal protection strategies should be considered for patients with preoperative renal insufficiency. Prehydration in the form of intravenous fluid administration serves as the primary prevention strategy for contrast-induced nephropathy.[20] The efficacy of intravenous sodium bicarbonate or N-acetylcysteine in the prevention of contrast-induced nephropathy remains unclear because of conflicting available evidence.[21] Nephrotoxic medications also should be avoided before contrast exposure. Adequate hydration managed by the anesthesia team takes into consideration the amount of preoperative renal dysfunction that exists, the complexity of the EVAR and expected amount of nephrotoxic dye, and the anticipated volume replacement necessary due to unanticipated blood loss.

Hemodynamic monitoring

Basic hemodynamic monitoring consists of pulmonary oximetry, capnography, urine output, temperature, and continuous arterial blood pressure monitoring. An intra-arterial catheter should be placed before induction of anesthesia on the contralateral side to any planned upper extremity surgical arterial access site. Complex EVARs, including those involving fenestrated or snorkel techniques with downward-angled visceral vessels, may require antegrade access via the axillosubclavian or brachial arteries to achieve cannulation of the visceral vessels or contralateral limb of the main body device. Large-bore intravenous access should be obtained given the potential for significant blood loss, particularly if a conversion to open surgery is indicated. Central venous access is not routinely required unless indicated by a patient's compromised baseline comorbid status or if a lengthy, complex endovascular intervention is anticipated.

Unlike open aortic surgery, blood loss during EVAR may be occult. Bleeding may occur at the level of the vascular access sites or may occur anywhere along the aorta or iliofemoral systems due to overly aggressive wire manipulation or the advancement of rigid stent graft deployment systems within small or heavily diseased vessels. Continuous monitoring of arterial blood pressure is therefore essential. The presence of abrupt unexplained hypotension should prompt immediate inspection of the vascular access sites followed by a thorough angiographic survey to search for potential sources of bleeding. Results of a multicenter trial comparing open versus endovascular AAA repair found that patients undergoing EVAR had a 60% reduction in intraoperative blood loss (650 mL) compared with those undergoing open repair (1600 mL). Moreover, blood transfusions were significantly less likely to be required in the EVAR group (12% vs 40% in open group). For even complicated EVAR, blood loss has been reasonable and still far less than open surgery. Many times, the adjunctive maneuvers, such as sewing iliac conduits or dealing with arm access, can increase blood loss associated with more complex EVAR.[22]

Anesthesia

Choice of anesthetic technique may be guided by hemodynamic status, baseline cardiopulmonary reserve, perioperative antiplatelet or anticoagulation usage, ability to lay flat, anticipated procedural duration, and patient preference. Brief periods of intermittent apnea are required during the course of the procedure to obtain optimal imaging quality in digital subtraction angiography. For that reason, laryngeal mask airway is often not a useful technique compared with endotracheal general anesthesia. As such, the patient's level of alertness and ability to perform intermittent breath-holds on command also should be considered. Lengthy procedures performed in awake patients may be associated with the development of restlessness or lower extremity ischemic symptoms owing to prolonged iliofemoral arterial occlusion. Such cases may compromise the safety of the operation or imaging quality, therefore prompting the need for additional sedation or conversion to general anesthesia.

General anesthesia is frequently regarded as more practical than locoregional anesthesia in these settings for a variety of reasons, including easier blood pressure management, control of sustained breath-holds required during the procedure, comfort of securing the airway in the rare incidence that rupture or conversion to open surgery is required, and elimination of patient-related factors that may compromise the conduct of the procedure (eg, anxiety, restlessness, pain). Locoregional anesthesia, ranging from simple infiltration of local anesthetic to full neuraxial blockade, may be advantageous in select cases, with benefits of this technique including less pharmacologically mediated myocardial depression and the potential for decreased intensive care unit and hospital length of stay.

Results of 6009 elective EVAR procedures with general, regional, or local/monitored anesthesia care (MAC) in the American College of Surgeons National Surgical Quality Improvement Program database demonstrated general anesthesia to be associated with increased postoperative length of stay and pulmonary morbidity compared with spinal and local/MAC anesthesia.[23] More recently, a systematic review and meta-analysis analyzed 10 studies of 13,459 patients given general or local anesthesia after EVAR.[24] Despite increased age and burden of baseline cardiopulmonary comorbidity in the group of patients receiving local anesthesia, the local anesthesia group was reported to have shorter procedural times, decreased postoperative lengths of stay, and significantly fewer postoperative complications compared with those receiving general anesthesia. Furthermore, a retrospective review of 784 patients receiving regional anesthesia in the form of an inguinal field block for femoral artery exposure during EVAR found that such anesthetic technique was associated with 97.9% technical success and only a 1.4% conversion rate to general anesthesia.[25] These data indicate that increasing the use of less-invasive anesthesia techniques is safe, feasible, and may ultimately serve as a primary strategy to significantly decrease the perioperative risk of patients undergoing EVAR. Also, given the development of increasingly lower-profile devices being used, the potential for blood loss and likelihood of a percutaneous approach minimizes unexpected complications and often allows for performing EVAR in the awake, cooperative patient. Nonagenarians are even not prohibitive, and results have been acceptable again in well-chosen patients.[26]

POSTPROCEDURE CARE

After an uncomplicated EVAR, patients are generally admitted overnight for the purposes of observation, continuation of intravenous fluid resuscitation, analgesia, and monitoring of groin access-sites. Complex EVARs or those performed in severely debilitated patients may necessitate a higher level of care, initiation of blood products, or early postoperative cross-sectional imaging. A recent report has noted that ambulatory percutaneous EVAR is feasible and safe in one-third of patients undergoing elective EVAR who did not have excessive medical risk, had good functional capacity, and underwent an uneventful procedure.[27]

COMPLICATIONS

Endoleak

Incomplete exclusion of the aneurysm sac with continued perfusion is referred to as endoleak and occurs in 10% to 50 % of cases.[28] The presence of an endoleak may be associated with continued aneurysm expansion and risk of rupture over time. There are 4 types of endoleaks. Type I endoleaks are related to inadequate proximal or distal fixation of the stent-graft to the aortic wall. Such endoleaks often can be corrected by endovascular methods, including placement of an extender cuff or stent. Type II endoleaks are caused by retrograde perfusion of the aneurysm sac from aortic side branches, most commonly the inferior mesenteric artery or lumbar arteries, and do not typically require intervention in the absence of aneurysm sac enlargement. Type III endoleaks result from junctional separation of the modular components or fractures or holes involving the endograft. Although relatively infrequent with newer-generation devices, this form of endoleak may occur in up to 35% of cases in branched and fenestrated EVARs.[29] These cases can be treated effectively with extension of an additional stent into the visceral vessels. Last, type IV endoleaks are caused by porosity of the stent graft fabric; however, this form of endoleak is exceedingly rare with current-generation devices. Many times the secondary interventions to repair endoleaks are performed in an angiography suite setting under conscious sedation without the use of anesthesia staff.

Access Site-Related Complications

Access-site complications may range from a local groin hematoma, infection, or lymphocele to more serious arterial injuries, such as dissection, thrombosis, pseudoaneurysm, arteriovenous fistula formation, or vessel perforation or avulsion. The incidence of severe complications is quite low, less than 3%, and can be minimized by careful preoperative planning, proper device selection, and judicious use of surgical conduits.

Colonic Ischemia

The incidence of colonic ischemia after EVAR is roughly similar to the 1% to 3% incidence observed after open AAA repair.[30,31] Although colonic ischemia after open repair is frequently profound and associated with significantly increased perioperative mortality, bowel ischemia after EVAR is frequently less severe. The mechanism of colonic ischemia after EVAR is likely multifactorial and may be due to direct stent graft coverage of the vessels supplying blood flow to the colon, as well as dislodgement of atherothrombotic debris resulting in microembolization to the superior mesenteric artery, inferior mesenteric artery, renal arteries, hypogastric arteries, or lower extremity arterial beds. Minimizing wire manipulation within an aneurysm with extensive circumferential thrombus or atheroma decreases the potential for such microembolic events.

Spinal Cord Ischemia

Although spinal cord ischemia is a well-known complication of endovascular repair involving the thoracic aorta, the incidence of this potentially devastating neurologic complication after EVAR is 0.21%.[32] The development of spinal cord ischemia is believed to be a result of both microembolization and interruption in the spinal collateral network by coverage of the lumbar, middle sacral, and hypogastric arteries. Additional risk factors for spinal cord ischemia as a result of microembolization into collateral vessels supplying the spinal cord include prolonged procedural time and extensive wire and catheter manipulation. Blood pressure augmentation and lumbar cerebrospinal fluid drainage represent the mainstays of treatment for spinal cord ischemia. Preoperative planning and recognition of the need for extensive aortic coverage, particularly in cases involving snorkel or fenestrated stent-grafts, which accommodate more proximal sealing zones, should prompt consideration for close neurologic monitoring, maintenance of a higher perioperative arterial blood pressure, and the potential for prophylactic lumbar drainage. Many centers, including our own, are quite aggressive about lumbar drains when there is anticipated coverage of the paravisceral segment or key collaterals in the spinal circulation. Lack of internal iliac flow or coverage of the subclavian artery during previous thoracic endovascular repair are additional risk factors for spinal cord ischemia.

Contrast-Induced Nephropathy

According to a recent nationwide survey, contrast-induced nephropathy occurs in 6.7% of cases.[33] The mean volume of contrast medium required during an EVAR case ranges between 50 and 100 mL. As previously stated, prevention of contrast-induced nephropathy is primarily focused on adequate hydration during and after the procedure. Sodium bicarbonate and N-acetylcysteine also are used regularly, although with less literature supporting their routine use. Additional approaches to minimize risk of contrast-induced nephropathy include performing EVAR under the guidance of intravascular ultrasound and, in some cases, using carbon dioxide as an alternative contrast medium.[34,35]

Post–Stent Implantation Syndrome

Endothelial activation by manipulation of the stent graft may lead to an inflammatory response manifested clinically by the presence of fever, increased inflammatory markers (eg, C-reactive protein), and leukocytosis without evidence of infection.

Duration of this inflammatory state is generally limited to 2 to 10 days and responds to nonsteroidal anti-inflammatory medication.

FUTURE CONSIDERATIONS/SUMMARY

In summary, the advent of EVAR, as it has replaced open surgery for routine and many times even complex aneurysm repair, has significant ramifications for the anesthesia team. Considerations of type of anesthesia, monitoring, risk assessment, and adjunctive procedures all need to be carefully discussed and planned. The success of this less-invasive technique has encouraged further refinement and miniaturization of the device components, as well as modifications to technical aspects, all rendering a theoretical advantage to the patient. That being said, these patients are still physiologically ill, and approaching these cases from an anesthesia standpoint without careful consideration can be problematic.

REFERENCES

1. Parodi JC, Palmaz JC, Barone HD. Transfemoral intraluminal graft implantation for abdominal aortic aneurysms. Ann Vasc Surg 1991;5:491–9.
2. Eidt JF, Mills J, Rhodes RS, et al. Comparison of surgical operative experience of trainees and practicing vascular surgeons: a report from the Vascular Surgery Board of the American Board of Surgery. J Vasc Surg 2011;53:1130–9.
3. Ullery BW, Nathan DP, Jackson BM, et al. Qualitative impact of the endovascular era on vascular surgeons' comfort level and enjoyment with open and endovascular AAA repairs. Vasc Endovascular Surg 2012;46:150–6.
4. Lederle FA, Freischlag JA, Kyriakides TC, et al. Outcomes following endovascular vs open repair of abdominal aortic aneurysm: a randomized trial. JAMA 2009; 302:1535–42.
5. Prinssen M, Verhoeven EL, Buth J, et al. A randomized trial comparing conventional and endovascular repair of abdominal aortic aneurysms. N Engl J Med 2004;351:1607–18.
6. Blankensteijn JD, de Jong SE, Prinssen M, et al. Two-year outcomes after conventional or endovascular repair of abdominal aortic aneurysms. N Engl J Med 2005; 352:2398–405.
7. Greenhalgh RM, Brown LC, Kwong GP, et al. Comparison of endovascular aneurysm repair with open repair in patients with abdominal aortic aneurysm (EVAR trial 1), 30-day operative mortality results: randomised controlled trial. Lancet 2004;364:843–8.
8. Brown LC, Powell JT. Risk factors for aneurysm rupture in patients kept under ultrasound surveillance. UK Small Aneurysm Trial Participants. Ann Surg 1999;230: 289–96.
9. Steyerberg EW, Kievit J, de Mol Van Otterloo JC, et al. Perioperative mortality of elective abdominal aortic aneurysm surgery. A clinical prediction rule based on literature and individual patient data. Arch Intern Med 1995;155:1998–2004.
10. Winterborn RJ, Amin I, Lyratzopoulos G, et al. Preferences for endovascular (EVAR) or open surgical repair among patients with abdominal aortic aneurysms under surveillance. J Vasc Surg 2009;49:576–81.
11. Lee JT, Ullery BW, Zarins CK, et al. EVAR deployment in anatomically challenging necks outside the IFU. Eur J Vasc Endovasc Surg 2013;46:65–73.
12. Arko FR, Filis KA, Seidel SA, et al. How many patients with infrarenal aneurysms are candidates for endovascular repair? The Northern California experience. J Endovasc Ther 2004;11:33–40.

13. Armerding MD, Rubin GD, Beaulieu CF, et al. Aortic aneurysmal disease: assessment of stent-graft treatment-CT versus conventional angiography. Radiology 2000;215:138–46.
14. Cuypers PW, Laheij RJ, Buth J. Which factors increase the risk of conversion to open surgery following endovascular abdominal aortic aneurysm repair? The EUROSTAR collaborators. Eur J Vasc Endovasc Surg 2000;20:183–9.
15. Fleisher LA, Beckman JA, Brown KA, et al. ACC/AHA 2007 guidelines on perioperative cardiovascular evaluation and care for noncardiac surgery: a report of the American College of Cardiology/American Heart Association Task Force on Practice Guidelines (Writing Committee to Revise the 2002 Guidelines on Perioperative Cardiovascular Evaluation for Noncardiac Surgery): developed in collaboration with the American Society of Echocardiography, American Society of Nuclear Cardiology, Heart Rhythm Society, Society of Cardiovascular Anesthesiologists, Society for Cardiovascular Angiography and Interventions, Society for Vascular Medicine and Biology, and Society for Vascular Surgery. Circulation 2007;116:e418–99.
16. Aziz IN, Lee JT, Kopchok GE, et al. Cardiac risk stratification in patients undergoing endoluminal graft repair of abdominal aortic aneurysm: a single-institution experience with 365 patients. J Vasc Surg 2003;38:56–60.
17. Browne TF, Hartley D, Purchas S, et al. A fenestrated covered suprarenal aortic stent. Eur J Vasc Endovasc Surg 1999;18:445–9.
18. Donas KP, Pecoraro F, Torsello G, et al. Use of covered chimney stents for pararenal aortic pathologies is safe and feasible with excellent patency and low incidence of endoleaks. J Vasc Surg 2012;55:659–65.
19. Mastracci TM, Greenberg RK, Eagleton MJ, et al. Durability of branches in branched and fenestrated endografts. J Vasc Surg 2013;57:926–33.
20. Weisbord SD, Palevsky PM. Prevention of contrast-induced nephropathy with volume expansion. Clin J Am Soc Nephrol 2008;3:273–80.
21. Sterling KA, Tehrani T, Rudnick MR. Clinical significance and preventive strategies for contrast-induced nephropathy. Curr Opin Nephrol Hypertens 2008;17:616–23.
22. Lee JT, Lee GK, Chandra V, et al. Early experience and lessons learned with fenestrated endografts compared to the snorkel/chimney technique. J Vasc Surg, in press.
23. Edwards MS, Andrews JS, Edwards AF, et al. Results of endovascular aortic aneurysm repair with general, regional, and local/monitored anesthesia care in the American College of Surgeons National Surgical Quality Improvement Program database. J Vasc Surg 2011;54:1273–82.
24. Karthikesalingam A, Thrumurthy SG, Young EL, et al. Locoregional anesthesia for endovascular aneurysm repair. J Vasc Surg 2012;56:510–9.
25. Setacci F, Sirignano P, Kamargianni V, et al. Inguinal field block for femoral artery exposure during endovascular aneurysm repair. J Endovasc Ther 2013;20:655–62.
26. Lee GK, Ullery BW, Lee JT. Elective EVAR in nonagenarians: Is there a survival benefit? Ann Vasc Surg, in press.
27. Dosluoglu HH, Lall P, Blochle R, et al. Ambulatory percutaneous endovascular abdominal aortic aneurysm repair. J Vasc Surg 2014;59:58–64.
28. Norwood MG, Lloyd GM, Bown MJ, et al. Endovascular abdominal aortic aneurysm repair. Postgrad Med J 2007;83:21–7.
29. Troisi N, Donas KP, Austermann M, et al. Secondary procedures after aortic aneurysm repair with fenestrated and branched endografts. J Endovasc Ther 2011;18:146–53.

30. Perry RJ, Martin MJ, Eckert MJ, et al. Colonic ischemia complicating open vs endovascular abdominal aortic aneurysm repair. J Vasc Surg 2008;48:272–7.
31. Becquemin JP, Kelley L, Zubilewicz T, et al. Outcomes of secondary interventions after abdominal aortic aneurysm endovascular repair. J Vasc Surg 2004;39:298–305.
32. Berg P, Kaufmann D, van Marrewijk CJ, et al. Spinal cord ischaemia after stent-graft treatment for infra-renal abdominal aortic aneurysms. Analysis of the Eurostar database. Eur J Vasc Endovasc Surg 2001;22:342–7.
33. Wald R, Waikar SS, Liangos O, et al. Acute renal failure after endovascular vs open repair of abdominal aortic aneurysm. J Vasc Surg 2006;43:460–6.
34. Chao A, Major K, Kumar SR, et al. Carbon dioxide digital subtraction angiography-assisted endovascular aortic aneurysm repair in the azotemic patient. J Vasc Surg 2007;45:451–8.
35. Gahlen J, Hansmann J, Schumacher H, et al. Carbon dioxide angiography for endovascular grafting in high-risk patients with infrarenal abdominal aortic aneurysms. J Vasc Surg 2001;33:646–9.

Postoperative ICU Management of Vascular Surgery Patients

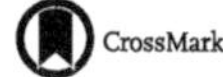

Ettore Crimi, MD[a,*], Charles C. Hill, MD[b]

KEYWORDS

- Critical care management • Vascular surgery • Thoracic aortic surgery
- Endovascular repair • Anesthetic management • Perioperative medical care

KEY POINTS

- Most patients undergoing major vascular procedures have multiple comorbidities and are at high risk for postoperative complications.
- Major postoperative complications affect multiple organ systems.
- Endovascular repair techniques may decrease mortality and morbidity in vascular surgical patients.

INTRODUCTION

Vascular surgery patients, whether undergoing open surgery or endovascular procedures, are at high risk for perioperative complications and require meticulous postoperative management. Widespread atherosclerotic disease, advanced age, and multiple comorbidities (often involving the cardiac, pulmonary, and renal organ systems), combined with the insult of major vascular surgery (which includes tissue damage, inflammatory responses, and profound hemodynamic changes), all serve to increase the risk of postoperative morbidity and mortality.

Preoperative risk stratification, careful perioperative management by the anesthesiologist, and scrupulous intensive care unit (ICU) care serve to minimize perioperative complications and optimize patient outcomes. Intraoperative anesthetic management should reestablish preoperative homeostasis and hemodynamics. Postoperative ICU management should support organ function until recovery from the surgical insult and provide early detection and effective management of postoperative complications.[1]

Funding Sources: None.
Conflict of Interest: None.

[a] Department of Anesthesia and Critical Care Medicine, Shands Hospital, University of Florida, 1600 Southwest Archer Road, PO Box 100254, Gainesville, FL 32610-025, USA; [b] Department of Anesthesia, Pain and Perioperative Medicine, Stanford University Medical Center, Stanford University School of Medicine, 300 Pasteur Drive, H3580, MC5640, Stanford, CA 94305, USA
* Corresponding author.
E-mail address: ecrimi@anest.ufl.edu

Anesthesiology Clin 32 (2014) 735–757
http://dx.doi.org/10.1016/j.anclin.2014.05.001 **anesthesiology.theclinics.com**
1932-2275/14/$ – see front matter

In this review, the authors discuss descending thoracic and thoracoabdominal aneurysms (TAAAs), abdominal aortic aneurysms (AAAs), and arterial occlusive disease, including carotid artery stenosis and peripheral artery disease (PAD), with an emphasis on the common postoperative complications and their critical care management.

AORTIC ANEURYSMS

Descending Thoracic Aneurysms and TAAAs: Open Repair

A descending thoracic aortic aneurysm involves any portion of the thoracic aorta distal to the left subclavian artery. TAAAs may extend from the left subclavian artery to different portions of the abdominal aorta, involving visceral arteries, such as the celiac axis, the superior mesenteric artery, and the renal arteries. **Fig. 1** demonstrates the Crawford classification system of TAAAs.

The incidence of diagnosed descending thoracic aneurysms and TAAAs is increasing as a result of improved radiographic imaging and an aging population and is estimated to be 10.4 per 100,000 people per year.[2] The common causes of thoracic aortic aneurysms are atherosclerotic degenerative disease, aortic dissection, and connective tissue diseases; less frequent causes are traumatic injury and infection.[3]

Open repair of TAAAs is the gold standard treatment.[4] Despite improvements in surgical techniques and perioperative care, the overall mortality ranges from 2% to 10%,

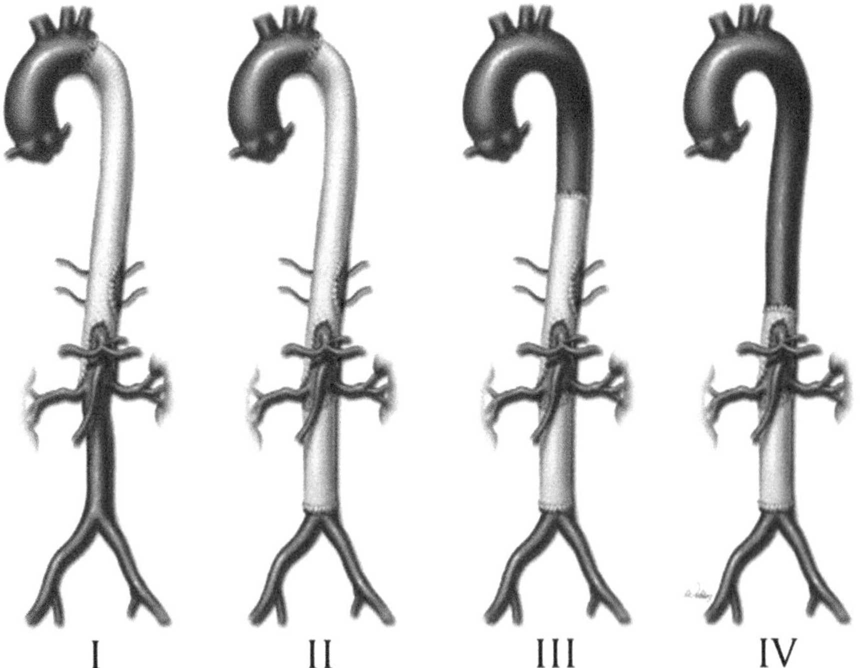

Fig. 1. Crawford classification of TAAA repairs. Extend I includes repairs of aorta from distal to the left subclavian artery to above the renal arteries. Extend II from distal to the left subclavian artery to the aortic bifurcation; Extend III from distal half of descending thoracic aorta to the aortic bifurcation. Extend IV involves most of the abdominal aorta from the diaphragm to the aortic bifurcation. (*From* Coselli JS, Bozinovski J, LeMaire SA. Open surgical repair of 2286 thoracoabdominal aortic aneurysms. Ann Thorac Surg 2007;83:S863; with permission.)

with better outcomes reported in high-volume thoracic aortic surgery centers. Mortality increases to more than 40% when emergent repair is required for acute dissection or rupture.[5] Preoperative renal dysfunction, intraoperative hypotension requiring large transfusions, postoperative paraplegia, and postoperative renal failure are associated with increased mortality.[6] These complications and other complications affecting the pulmonary, renal, neurologic, cardiac, gastrointestinal, and hematologic systems are discussed later (**Box 1**).[7,8]

Pulmonary complications

Postoperative respiratory complications are the most common sequelae of thoracoabdominal aortic surgery, occurring after approximately 30% of cases, and are associated with a high mortality rate and increased length of hospitalization.[9,10] Frequent respiratory complications include postoperative ventilation longer than 48 hours, atelectasis, pleural effusions, pneumonia, reintubation, and need for tracheostomy. Preoperative risk factors include a history of smoking and associated chronic obstructive pulmonary disease (COPD). Intraoperative risk factors include surgical division of the diaphragm, prolonged one-lung ventilation (OLV) (with left lung collapse

Box 1
Open TAAA repair: postoperative complications

- Pulmonary
  - Atelectasis
  - Pleural effusions
  - Pneumonia
  - Postoperative ventilation greater than 48 hours
  - Acute lung injury/acute respiratory distress syndrome
  - Tracheostomy
- Renal
  - Acute kidney injury
- Neurologic
  - Spinal cord ischemia
  - Stroke
- Cardiac
  - Myocardial ischemia
  - Congestive heart failure
  - Arrhythmias
- Hematologic
  - Bleeding
  - Thrombocytopenia
  - Heparin-induced thrombocytopenia
- Gastrointestinal
  - Mesenteric ischemia
  - Hepatic dysfunction
  - Biliary disease

and reexpansion, and potential right lung ventilator-induced lung injury), and massive blood product transfusion.[11]

Massive intraoperative fluid shifts often produce extensive facial and neck swelling that precludes the exchange of the double-lumen endotracheal tube for a standard single-lumen endotracheal tube. Prolonged postoperative use of a double-lumen endotracheal tube may also contribute to airway morbidity by increasing the risk of tracheal and proximal bronchial laceration or perforation.

A multimodal approach to the perioperative management of postsurgical patients has been shown to minimize pulmonary complications.[12] These approaches may be divided into the preoperative, intraoperative, and postoperative periods.

The primary preoperative strategy involves identifying those patients at highest risk for postoperative pulmonary complications. These patients are often tobacco smokers and may present with moderate to severe obstructive lung disease with a reduced forced expiratory volume in 1 second/forced vital capacity ratio and decreased carbon monoxide diffusing capacity. Occasionally, patients present with restrictive lung disease caused by interstitial lung disease, thoracic cage deformities, and neuromuscular disorders. Both of these high-risk populations require optimization of pulmonary function preoperatively, either through enhanced medical therapy or lifestyle changes, such as weight loss and smoking cessation.

Intraoperative anesthetic management plays a large role in determining patients' postoperative course. Evidence suggests that avoiding allogenic blood product transfusions reduces postoperative morbidity and mortality, which has resulted in the development of more conservative transfusion thresholds for hemoglobin levels in these patients (7 g/dL). Perioperative whole blood clotting (viscoelastic) measures like thromboelastography (TEG) help inform targeted factor and platelet replacements, thereby reducing allogenic blood product transfusions. Additionally, emerging evidence indicates that the use of lung-protective ventilator strategies may also provide some postoperative pulmonary benefit. Surgically, the preservation of phrenic nerve function and diaphragmatic integrity, especially in patients with COPD, reduces pulmonary morbidity.

Postoperative strategies focus on adequate volume resuscitation, rational pain management, and early extubation. In patients with normal left and right ventricular systolic function, volume resuscitation should be administered until there is return of preoperative hemodynamics. Euvolemia should be accompanied by a resolution of any lactic acidosis present on completion of the surgical procedure and transfer to the ICU. A bedside transthoracic echocardiogram (TTE) or transesophageal echocardiogram (TEE) should be performed to diagnose any unexplained hemodynamic perturbations. Invasive hemodynamic monitoring is beneficial in those patients with moderate to severe right or left ventricular systolic dysfunction, pulmonary hypertension, or ongoing myocardial ischemia.

Modern pain management uses multimodal therapy, including regional anesthesia and nonopioid analgesic adjuncts, and frequently allows for tracheal extubation in the operating room. Epidural opioids allow for early neurologic assessment of the lower extremities. If the procedure is too long or complex to allow for immediate extubation, these adjuncts may be continued in the ICU to optimize respiratory mechanics after the patients' trachea is extubated.

On arrival to the ICU, 30° head-up positioning, as part of ventilator-associated pneumonia (VAP) bundle, is very important and also serves to decrease facial edema. Active suctioning of blood clots from the endotracheal tube and prophylactic bronchoscopy before extubation often improves left lung functioning after a long intraoperative period of OLV. Early extubation allows for early patient mobilization, as does early removal of any left chest tubes, which in turn minimizes the risk of infection. Increased oxygen requirements (reflecting an increased A-a gradient) are common in the immediate postoperative period, with acute lung injury (ALI) and acute respiratory distress syndrome criteria often satisfied. Aggressive pulmonary toilet (incentive spirometry, intermittent positive-pressure ventilation) and early application of noninvasive positive-pressure ventilation are important tools in the arsenal to treat these clinical entities and to prevent early, postoperative pulmonary complications.

Application of nasal continuous positive airway pressure, with 10 cm H_2O immediately after extubation, has been associated with fewer pulmonary complications and reduced length of hospital stay. This effect is thought to occur by maintaining functional residual capacity, thus preventing atelectasis and hypoxemia, and reducing the work of breathing.[13] In patients with prolonged ventilator support, early tracheostomy can be beneficial for early mobilization and expedited transfer out of the ICU.[9]

Renal complications

Patients undergoing thoracoabdominal surgery are at high risk for developing postoperative acute kidney injury (AKI). Although various studies have used different criteria to define renal dysfunction, the incidence of postoperative AKI requiring dialysis ranges between 5% and 15%, and its occurrence is associated with a worse outcome.[14,15]

The most important preoperative predictors of AKI are preoperative renal dysfunction (chronic kidney disease [CKD]) and severity of atherosclerosis disease. Modifiable intraoperative risk factors include the duration of aortic cross-clamping, blood transfusion, and hemodynamic instability.[16] The pathophysiology of perioperative AKI is primarily the result of acute tubular necrosis and is exacerbated by perioperative hypotension, hypovolemia, atheromatous embolization, renal ischemia, and rhabdomyolysis.

Nephrotoxins, such as contrast agents, nonsteroidal antiinflammatory drugs, and aminoglycoside antibiotics, increase the risk of perioperative renal dysfunction. Intraoperative strategies for renal protection include minimizing renal ischemic time, using selective renal perfusion with cold protective solutions, and using distal aortic perfusion techniques.[17,18] Intraoperative use of multiple pharmacologic agents (renal-dose dopamine, loop diuretics, mannitol, N-acetylcysteine, fenoldopam) has failed to demonstrate significant clinical benefit.[19]

Perioperative maintenance of adequate intravascular volume and renal perfusion pressure, while limiting exposure to nephrotoxic medications remains the most effective approach for minimizing postoperative renal dysfunction. With the onset of renal failure, meticulous management of fluids, electrolytes, and acid-base status is imperative; renal replacement therapy should be instituted promptly when clinically indicated.

Neurologic complications

Spinal cord ischemia Spinal cord ischemia (SCI) resulting in paraparesis or paralysis is the most feared and devastating complication of thoracoabdominal aortic surgery. Advances in spinal protection strategies have significantly reduced the incidence of SCI to a current rate of 2% to 8%.[7,20,21] The risk factors include the extent of the aneurysm (7.8% incidence of SCI in type II TAAA), aortic dissection, emergent surgery, perioperative hypotension or hypoxemia, and duration of aortic cross-clamp time (27% incidence with ischemic time >60 minutes, 8% incidence with ischemic time <30 minutes).[8,22]

SCI may present with an immediate deficit at the end of the procedure or on awakening in the ICU, but it may also present after days to weeks. SCI deficits often resolve or improve over time with aggressive physical therapy and rehabilitation but are dense and permanent in the worst cases. SCI typically presents as an anterior spinal artery syndrome with loss of motor function and pain and temperature sensation. Proprioception and vibratory sensation may be preserved in one or both lower extremities. The severity of the motor deficit can range from flaccid paraplegia to varying degrees of paraparesis, as described by the modified Tarlov scale (**Table 1**).[23]

The anterior spinal cord is supplied by the anterior spinal artery, a single vessel reinforced by a succession of radicular arteries, the most important usually being the artery of Adamkiewicz, which originates in the area between the T9 and T12 vertebral bodies in most individuals. Spinal cord perfusion pressure (SCPP) is determined by the difference between mean arterial pressure (MAP) and cerebrospinal fluid (CSF) pressure or the central venous pressure (CVP), whichever is greater.

SCPP = MAP − CSF pressure (or CVP)

Aortic cross-clamping may lead to SCI by decreasing distal MAP, which decreases distal perfusion pressure to the spinal cord and increases CSF pressure by increasing CVP and CSF production. SCI may be further exacerbated intraoperatively if transection of major anterior spinal arteries and intercostal/lumbar arteries combines with hypotension to compromise blood supply and oxygen delivery to the spinal cord.

Ischemia and reperfusion trigger the release of neurotoxins (free radicals, excitatory neurotransmitters, and nitric oxide), which amplify and propagate SCI and may potentiate progression to infarction.[24] Intraoperative perfusion strategies to prevent or mitigate SCI include minimizing spinal cord ischemic time while providing distal aortic perfusion via left heart bypass or partial or total cardiopulmonary bypass (with or without deep hypothermic circulatory arrest). Surgically, preserving the blood supply with reattachment of critical intercostal arteries may reduce postoperative SCI.

The primary objective of intraoperative and postoperative hemodynamic management is to ensure a MAP greater than 90 mm Hg and an optimized cardiac index with the lowest appropriate CVP. Attenuating ischemic injury to the spinal cord using hypothermia, barbiturates, steroids, naloxone, or free radical scavengers are frequently used therapeutic adjuncts in the intraoperative and postoperative management of these patients. However, despite some scant data supporting the use of naloxone in this setting, hypothermia is the only adjunct with documented clinical efficacy. Monitoring spinal cord function with motor-evoked potentials and somatosensory-evoked potentials has also shown potential in reducing the incidence of postoperative SCI.[25–27]

Early neurologic assessment in the immediate postoperative period is essential for prompt recognition of SCI. Immediate intervention includes optimizing hemodynamic status and using aggressive CSF drainage to reduce CSF pressure to 7 to 8 mm Hg. These initial maneuvers enhance spinal cord perfusion and often restore neurologic function.[28,29]

Table 1
Modified Tarlov scale

Scale	Motor Function	Deficit
0	No lower extremity movement	Paraplegia
1	Lower extremity motion without gravity	Paraplegia
2	Lower extremity motion against gravity	Paraplegia
3	Able to stand with assistance	Paraparesis
4	Able to walk with assistance	Paraparesis
5	Normal	Normal

Adequate cardiac output may be maintained by optimizing fluid status or by initiating chronotropes or inotropes to maximize cardiac function and performance. The hemoglobin level should be increased to 10 mg/dL to maximize oxygen delivery to the ischemic spinal cord tissue. TEE or invasive hemodynamic monitoring with a pulmonary artery catheter (PAC) is extremely beneficial in these settings. Afterload augmentation (with either alpha-adrenergic agonists or vasopressin) is also appropriate when all other parameters have been optimized and the goal MAP of 90 to 100 mm Hg has not been achieved.

Lumbar CSF drainage improves spinal perfusion pressure by decreasing CSF pressure. CSF drainage using a lumbar drain has been shown to reduce the risk of SCI and can improve or reverse a postoperative neurologic deficit.[30–32] CSF drainage should be started intraoperatively and is typically maintained for 72 hours with a CSF pressure goal less than 10 mm Hg. Any clinical sign of a neurologic deficit should be treated by decreasing the CSF target pressure to less than 5 mm Hg. Placement of a lumbar drain after the onset of paralysis may reverse delayed-onset SCI (**Table 2**).[33–35]

Overaggressive CSF drainage can precipitate intracranial bleeding.[36] A judicious drainage rate (less than 15 mL/h in neurologically intact patients) is recommended.[37] Placement of an 18-G Tuohy needle for the lumbar drain may result in the formation of a spinal cord hematoma with cord compression and paraplegia.[36] A high index of clinical suspicion, combined with frequent physical examinations and neurologic checks, often leads to early diagnosis and prompt diagnostic radiographic imaging. Surgical decompression within 8 hours of the onset of symptoms is key to achieving resolution of neurologic deficits.

Cerebrovascular vascular accident Cerebrovascular accident (CVA) occurs in 3% to 10% of patients following thoracic aortic surgery.[38] Ischemic CVA is mainly caused by embolic injury from atheromatous disease and subsequent hypoperfusion. Age, dissection, extensive aortic atheroma, and emergent repair are associated with an increased risk of perioperative CVA. The diagnostic workup with computed tomography (CT) and magnetic resonance imaging (MRI) (lumbar drain catheters are MRI compatible, whereas spring-wound epidural catheters are not) should occur promptly whenever there is clinical suspicion of CVA. Postoperative care should focus on preventing secondary brain injury by maintaining adequate cerebral perfusion pressure while avoiding hyperthermia and hyperglycemia.[39] When clinically indicated, a hypothermic cooling protocol and consultation with a neurocritical care intensivist should be promptly used.

Cardiovascular complications

Cardiovascular complications occur in 10% to 20% of patients and include myocardial ischemia, congestive heart failure, and arrhythmias (primarily atrial fibrillation).[8,22]

Table 2
Treatment of spinal cord ischemia

Organ System	Treatment Intervention
Neurologic	↓ CSF pressure to 5 mm Hg (insert lumbar drain if delayed-onset spinal cord injury)
Cardiovascular	Maintain MAP 90–100 mm Hg Augment cardiac output maximally Ensure adequate DO_2 Decrease CVP if >10 mm Hg
Hematologic	Maintain hemoglobin 10 g/dL

Abbreviation: DO_2, oxygen delivery.

Uncontrolled hypertension can exacerbate postoperative bleeding and compromise suture lines. Hypertension and tachycardia also increase myocardial oxygen demand through increased ventricular wall tension and myocardial work, which exposes high-risk patients to an increased risk of myocardial ischemia and ventricular dysfunction.

Prolonged hypotension can aggravate end-organ dysfunction through inadequate perfusion pressure and oxygen supply. Many investigators recommend a target systolic blood pressure within 20% of patients' baseline; appropriate hemodynamic monitoring using PAC, TTE, or TEE is strongly encouraged in these high-risk patients. TTE or TEE may demonstrate ventricular wall motion abnormalities indicating myocardial ischemia before changes appear on the electrocardiogram (ECG).

Fluid management requires attention to detail, especially on the second and third postoperative days, when third-space fluid mobilization tends to occur. If indicated, gentle diuresis may be initiated to decrease the risk of volume overload and avoid hypoxia, pulmonary edema, and hypertension. Postoperative beta-blockade and continuation of 3-hydroxy-3-methylglutaryl–coenzyme A reductase inhibitor medications (statins) have been shown to exhibit cardioprotective effects in this patient population.[40,41] Postoperative antiplatelet therapy (usually aspirin) should be started as soon as the risk of bleeding is acceptably low.

Hematologic complications

Postoperative hemorrhage occurs in 2% to 5% of patients after thoracic aortic surgery and may require surgical re-exploration, further increasing morbidity and mortality.[42] Extensive surgical dissection, major intraoperative blood loss and subsequent massive blood transfusion, systemic heparinization, mesenteric ischemia, and hypothermia combine to produce a dilutional and consumptive coagulopathy.[43–45] Persistent postoperative bleeding requires prompt and aggressive treatment, including strict blood pressure control to minimize risk of the bleeding, and correction of hypothermia, acidosis, and hypocalcemia.

Treatment with blood components should not be delayed in order to prevent further depletion of coagulation factors and platelets. Ideally, replacement of clotting factors, platelets, and fibrinogen should be guided by standard coagulation tests (prothrombin time/international normalized ratio, partial thromboplastin time, and fibrinogen) along with real-time whole blood viscoelastic results, by using TEG or rotational thromboelastometry (ROTEM).[46] In the absence of active bleeding and acute myocardial ischemia, or concern for SCI, a restrictive transfusion strategy to maintain hemoglobin at more than 7 g/dL is recommended for all patients without significant underlying coronary artery disease (CAD).[47,48] When clinical evidence for transfusion is equivocal, serial monitoring of central venous or mixed venous oxygen saturation provides an excellent assessment of tissue oxygen delivery.

In the early postoperative period, thrombocytopenia may occur secondary to platelet consumption in the setting of persistent bleeding or sequestration by aortic graft material. Less commonly, the development of heparin-dependent, platelet-activating antibodies may cause heparin-induced thrombocytopenia (HIT). HIT should always be considered in thrombocytopenic patients recently exposed to heparin. Later in the postoperative course, thrombocytosis and decreased fibrinolysis with hyperfibrinogenemia promote a hypercoagulable state with increased risk of thrombotic complications, requiring institution of anticoagulation (eg, low-molecular-weight heparin).[49]

Gastrointestinal complications

Mesenteric ischemia is a potentially fatal complication of thoracic aortic surgery, with an incidence of 2% and very high mortality, usually higher than 60%.[50] Splanchnic hypoperfusion and ischemia may occur secondary to embolic, thrombotic, or mechanical obstruction (such as occurs when an aortic dissection flap produces a static or dynamic obstruction to the ostia of a visceral blood vessel) of arterial inflow. Clinical evidence of abdominal pain with a persistent lactic acidosis is often an early warning sign. Mesenteric ischemia triggers a systemic inflammatory response with distant organ damage and often worsens any previously ongoing coagulopathy. To prevent unfavorable outcomes, it is absolutely essential to perform serial abdominal examinations with early general surgery consultation and timely radiographic evaluation.

Postoperative hepatic dysfunction and biliary disease occur in 1.6% and 0.3% of patients, respectively, and are associated with increased mortality.[50]

Ileus, pancreatitis, cholecystitis, and ischemic colitis may have also been seen following open TAAA repair. These conditions are also commonly seen following open repair of AAAs and are discussed in more detail later.

Descending Thoracic Aneurysms and TAAAs: Endovascular Repair

In the last 20 years, thoracic endovascular aortic repair (TEVAR) has emerged as a less invasive and potentially safer alternative to open surgical repair.[51] Although TEVAR was initially limited to patients considered at high risk for conventional open surgical repair, the evolution of aortic stent graft (endograft) design and delivery techniques has expanded its application. Currently, endovascular stent grafting can be applied to elective and emergent repair of TAAAs, pseudoaneurysms, complicated type-B aortic dissections, and traumatic aortic injuries as long as the technical criteria for deployment of the stent are satisfied.[52]

The procedure involves the delivery and deployment of one or more self-expanding aortic grafts within the aorta under fluoroscopic guidance, through percutaneous access via the femoral artery or, less frequently, the iliac artery. Fenestrated and branched stent grafts are used to maintain perfusion of the visceral arteries that originate from the covered aortic segment.

Hybrid procedures, which combine open surgery and endovascular stenting, use the creation of an extra-anatomical bypass to the branch arteries of the aorta and expand the indications for endovascular stenting.[53] An open left carotid-subclavian bypass is recommended to prevent upper extremity ischemia in patients who need elective TEVAR when the proximal seal requires covering the ostium of the left subclavian artery and in selected patients with anatomy that may compromise perfusion to the brain, spinal cord, and heart.[54]

Endovascular repair avoids extensive aortic dissection and aortic cross-clamping and is generally associated with reduced blood loss, less postoperative pain, and a shorter recovery period. A recent meta-analysis demonstrated a significant reduction in 30-day mortality, stroke, SCI, and cardiopulmonary complications for endovascular repair as compared with open surgery. Higher rates of graft-related complications and a larger number of reinterventions were seen in the endovascular group, and no differences in late mortality were found between the 2 groups.[55] Endovascular stent grafting is not without risks, and complications can be immediate or delayed (beyond 1 year) (**Box 2**).[56,57]

Early complications of TEVAR include vascular access injuries, stroke, SCI, and AKI.

Vascular access injury occurs in 15% to 20% of TEVAR cases. The large delivery catheters require the presence of an adequately sized femoral or iliac artery. Prosthetic conduits or alternative sites are required in 20% of patients. Frequent injuries include iliofemoral lacerations and rupture, pseudoaneurysm formation and retroperitoneal hematoma. Lower extremity ischemia is another significant complication and usually presents with a decreased or absent distal pulse on the operative side.

Box 2
Early complications of TEVAR

Vascular access injury (15%–20%)

Stroke (2%–8%)

SCI (3%–10%)

AKI (2%)

Postimplantation syndrome

Stroke occurs in roughly 2% to 8% of TEVAR procedures and is typically an embolic event, with distributions in both hemispheres of the anterior and posterior circulations. Risk and severity of stroke are related to the severity and extent of atherosclerotic disease within the aorta, along with the degree and duration of wire or catheter instrumentation. History of prior stroke, CT grade IV atheroma (>5 mm) in the aortic arch, chronic renal insufficiency, proximal descending aorta coverage, and long descending thoracic aorta segment coverage all increase the risk of stroke.[58]

SCI occurs in 3% to 10% of cases in the setting of TEVAR and may present as immediate or delayed. The factors that contribute to an increased risk of SCI include length of thoracic aorta coverage (thereby leading to exclusion of intercostal arteries at the T6 to T12 vertebral levels, which supply the anterior spinal artery); prior AAA repair (which compromises pelvic and hypogastric collateral vessels); pelvic occlusive atherosclerotic disease; perioperative hypotension (with SCPP <70 mm Hg); severe atherosclerotic disease; perioperative renal failure; and subclavian artery coverage.[59,60]

CSF drainage should begin intraoperatively and continue through the initial 72-hour postoperative period, similar to open TAAA repair. Postoperative placement should be considered as a rescue maneuver for delayed SCI.[61] The primary goals of SCI management in the ICU after TEVAR are identical to the management used after open TAAA repair, discussed previously.

AKI is seen after approximately 2% of TEVAR procedures. Embolism, hypoperfusion, and contrast-induced nephropathy all may cause AKI. Identified predictors of AKI are preoperative renal dysfunction, blood transfusion, and extent of aortic disease.[62] Perioperative strategies that may reduce the incidence of AKI should be strongly considered in medium- to high-risk patients and include maintaining adequate renal perfusion pressure, using iso-osmolar nonionic contrast, intravenous bicarbonate infusion, preoperative acetylcysteine administration, and avoiding nephrotoxic agents.[63]

Postimplantation syndrome is frequently seen after TEVAR and includes mild leukocytosis, fever, and elevation of C-reactive protein. This clinical syndrome is thought to be secondary to a significant inflammatory response, resulting in endothelial activation by the endoprosthesis. Postimplantation syndrome is associated with large segment coverage and the use of multiple stent devices.

Late complications include stent graft migration, endoleaks with aneurysm expansion and rupture, stent graft infection, and erosion into the esophagus. The potential for these long-term, late complications requires long-term surveillance of the aorta. Endoleak, defined as persistent blood flow outside the lumen of the endoprosthesis and within the aneurysm sac following endovascular graft stenting, can occur in up to 30% of cases. Endoleaks are usually classified into 5 types. Types I and III are considered risk factors for aneurysm enlargement and rupture and require intervention to eliminate the leak (**Box 3**).[64]

Box 3
Late complications of TEVAR

Stent graft migration

Endoleak with aneurysm expansion and rupture

Stent graft infection

Esophageal erosion

AAA: Open Repair

AAA occurs in 5% to 10% of men aged more than 65 years. Smoking, male gender, and age are the predominant risk factors. Most AAAs involves the infrarenal aorta. Elective, open repair may be performed via either a transabdominal or retroperitoneal approach and carries a 5% mortality, with 30% of patients experiencing one or more major postoperative complications. The risk of postoperative complications is directly correlated with increasing procedure duration and site of aortic cross-clamping. Operative mortality for a ruptured AAA approximates 50%, and these patients frequently experience a prolonged and complicated ICU course (**Box 4**).[65]

Pulmonary complications

Major postoperative pulmonary complications occur in 16% to 18 % of patients after open AAA repair, with a higher incidence for emergent cases, and are associated with increased mortality.[66,67] Preoperatively, a history of cigarette smoking with coexisting COPD or other intrinsic lung disease confers a higher risk of postoperative pulmonary complications. Intraoperative risk factors include a long aortic cross-clamp time and large blood loss requiring massive volume transfusion. Fluid sequestration and abdominal distension are adverse sequelae that lead to compromised respiratory mechanics and prolonged mechanical ventilation. In extubated patients, these preoperative and intraoperative risk factors combine to hinder effective pulmonary toilet and increase the risk of postoperative atelectasis, pneumonia, and reintubation.[68,69]

Box 4
Open AAA repair: postoperative complications

Pulmonary

Cardiac

- Myocardial ischemia/infarction
- Postoperative hemorrhage
- Lower extremity ischemia

Gastrointestinal

- Ileus
- Pancreatitis
- Cholecystitis
- Ischemic colitis
- Abdominal compartment syndrome

Renal

- AKI

Preoperative identification of high-risk patients with severe lung disease (assessed by room air arterial blood gas and pulmonary function tests) allows for optimization of medical therapy and preoperative training in incentive spirometry and deep-breathing maneuvers.[12,70] Postoperatively, adequate pain management using a multimodal approach, early extubation, and respiratory physiotherapy can reduce major pulmonary complications.[71] In patients who require prolonged mechanical ventilation, inspiratory muscle strength training can help in weaning from the ventilator.[72]

Cardiovascular complications

Myocardial infarction Patients with AAAs have a high prevalence of CAD and experience a 15% risk of cardiac complications. Two different types of postoperative myocardial infarction (MI) occur: an early MI, occurring from the end of surgery to 12 to 24 hours postoperatively, and a delayed MI, typically presenting 24 to 72 hours postoperatively. Early MIs present with a sudden onset and are likely caused by an acute coronary occlusion from a rupture of a vulnerable plaque. Delayed MIs are often preceded by a period of myocardial ischemia secondary to an imbalance between myocardial oxygen supply and demand.[73]

Postoperative serial ECGs and troponin measurement are strongly recommended for early detection of myocardial ischemia in medium- to high-risk patients. Postoperative MI should be aggressively treated with beta-blockers for heart rate control, antiplatelet drugs, statins, adequate analgesia, and supplemental oxygenation.[74] Perioperative beta-blocker administration in patients at high risk for perioperative myocardial ischemia has significant beneficial effects,[75–77] although their use in patients with few or no risk factors, and to a fixed systolic blood pressure target without consideration of initial preoperative values, can increase the risk of death from noncardiac causes and stroke.[78,79] Statins, in combination with beta-blockers, decrease perioperative mortality in vascular surgery patients,[41] whereas their acute withdrawal significantly increases the risk of perioperative myocardial ischemia.[80]

Postoperative hemorrhage Bleeding from disruption of aortic graft anastomoses is a major surgical concern after open AAA repair. Strict blood pressure control is imperative until the risk of surgical postoperative hemorrhage is low enough to allow for a return to the patients' preoperative hemodynamic profile. When massive red blood cell transfusion is required, a resuscitation approach using fresh frozen plasma is beneficial in reducing intravascular depletion of clotting factors. Laboratory values of objective parameters from clotting assessments, such as TEG, are beneficial in guiding blood product administration therapy.

Lower extremity ischemia Lower extremity ischemia as result of distal atheromatous emboli can occur in 2% to 5% of patients after open AAA repair. Frequent lower extremities perfusion assessment via Doppler ultrasound is extremely helpful in promptly detecting this potential surgical emergency.

Gastrointestinal complications

Ileus The extensive mobilization of viscera, together with the frequent sacrifice of the inferior mesenteric artery during open aneurysm repair, increases the risk of postoperative gastrointestinal complications. All patients experience a mild ileus, whereas prolonged postoperative ileus occurs in 10% to 15% of patients. Removing the nasogastric tube early to decrease the incidence of respiratory complications and instituting early feeding have been advocated after AAA repair,[81] but caution should be taken until clinical evidence of bowel function has returned.

Pancreatitis and cholecystitis Pancreatitis, as result of direct trauma, ischemia, or acalculous cholecystitis, may also occur postoperatively. Pancreatitis from trauma and manipulation is usually self-limited. In severe cases, acalculous cholecystitis may require percutaneous cholecystotomy or surgical cholecystectomy.

Ischemic colitis Ischemic colitis is a rare complication (incidence of 0.6%) with a high mortality rate (40%–65%). The exclusion of the inferior mesenteric artery leaves the descending colon, sigmoid colon, and rectum dependent on collateral flow. Suprarenal aortic cross-clamping, prolonged cross-clamp time, and extensive atherosclerotic disease increase the risk of this highly fatal complication. Typically, patients will experience bloody diarrhea and increasing abdominal pain. Laboratory results reveal leukocytosis and progressive lactic acidosis on the first or second postoperative day.

The diagnosis is confirmed by sigmoidoscopy or colonoscopy.[82] Patients with transmural colonic necrosis require exploratory laparotomy with resection of the involved segment and diverting colostomy, whereas patients with reversible mucosal ischemia are treated with bowel rest and broad-spectrum antibiotics.

Abdominal compartment syndrome Massive fluids resuscitation, especially after emergent repair of a ruptured AAA, increases the risk of intra-abdominal hypertension (IAH) (normal intra-abdominal pressure measured by bladder pressure is <12 mm Hg).[83] The deleterious effects of IAH extends beyond the damage of the intra-abdominal organs (bowel, renal, and liver ischemia) affecting the cardiovascular (decreased venous return, increased afterload, changes in ventricular compliance), respiratory (decreased chest wall compliance and function residual capacity, increased peak and plateau pressures), and central venous systems (increased intracranial pressure and decreased cerebral perfusion pressure). Intra-abdominal pressure should be checked on arrival of patients in the ICU; if it is elevated, serial measurements should be started. An intra-abdominal pressure more than 20 mm Hg associated with evidence of new organ failure defines abdominal compartment syndrome and requires aggressive medical management and possible early surgical decompression.[84]

Renal complications

AKI The incidence of AKI after infrarenal AAA repair is 5%, with dialysis required in less than 0.6% of cases. AKI after suprarenal aortic cross-clamping approaches 15%. Aortic cross-clamping reduces renal blood flow by 45% with infrarenal clamping and by up to 80% with suprarenal clamping. A concomitant increase in renal vascular resistance and redistribution of flow toward the cortical layers follows, predisposing the renal medulla to ischemic injury.[85,86]

Perioperatively, maintenance of adequate intravascular volume and renal perfusion pressure during and after aortic cross-clamping are paramount in mitigating postoperative renal dysfunction. No pharmacologic strategies have been proven to confer a significant beneficial clinical effect; therefore, avoiding nephrotoxins and hypovolemic hypotension are the primary objectives of postoperative critical care management.[19]

AAA: Endovascular Aortic Repair

In appropriate patients, elective and emergent AAA repairs can be performed using an endovascular approach.[87–89] In the United States, nearly 60% of AAAs are electively repaired by endovascular aortic repair (EVAR),[90] which is less invasive than open surgical repair and has been associated with a lower 30 day-mortality and morbidity when compared with open repair.[91,92] Postoperative EVAR complications are similar to those observed after TEVAR, with a reduced incidence of stroke and SCI.

ARTERIAL OCCLUSIVE DISEASE

Carotid Artery Stenosis

Stroke represents one of the major causes of mortality and long-term disability in the United States. Approximately 66% of strokes are caused by thromboembolic events, and atherosclerosis of the extracranial internal carotid artery (ICA) is the major risk factor.[93] Carotid endarterectomy (CEA) is recommended for symptomatic patients with ICA stenosis of 50% to 99% and asymptomatic patients with ICA stenosis of 60% to 99%.[94]

CEA involves a longitudinal neck incision along the anterior border of the sternocleidomastoid muscle, with exposure of the common carotid artery and ICA. The carotid artery is cross-clamped, and a shunt may be placed to bypass the clamped portion of the carotid artery to preserve blood flow to the brain. An endarterectomy is performed, and patch angioplasty of the diseased portion of the artery is completed under general or regional anesthesia.[95]

Carotid artery stenting has emerged as a less invasive procedure and is typically reserved for symptomatic patients with ICA stenosis of 50% to 99% who are at a high risk for traditional open CEA.[94] Neurologic monitoring is essential after open CEA or carotid stenting for early detection of any signs or symptoms of neurologic complications (**Box 5**).

Neurologic complications

Stroke (CVA) Postoperative CVA is a highly morbid complication, with an incidence of 0.25% to 7.0% following CEA. Neurologic deficits may be immediately evident postoperatively or may present 12 to 24 hours after surgery. Embolism, thrombosis, hemorrhage, hypoperfusion, and hypotension may result in a CVA either independently or in combination. Any changes or defects noted in the neurologic examination require rapid diagnostic investigation to evaluate patency of the carotid arteries (duplex ultrasound, CT/CT angiography of the brain, arteriography) and potential re-exploration.

If surgical correction is not required, standard critical care management of stroke should be instituted, including neurocritical care consultation and radiographic imaging, and electroencephalography monitoring if seizures are suspected. Cerebral perfusion pressure should be maintained via support of MAP after hemorrhagic CVA has been ruled out.

Box 5
Carotid endarterectomy: postoperative complications

- Neurologic
  - Stroke (CVA)
  - Cerebral hyperperfusion syndrome
  - Cranial nerve injury
- Cardiac
  - Myocardial ischemia
  - Postoperative hypertension
  - Postoperative hypotension
- Pulmonary
  - Upper airway compromise
  - Hypercarbia
  - Hypoxemia

Cerebral hyperperfusion syndrome Cerebral hyperperfusion syndrome occurs in 1% to 2% of patients following CEA and usually presents 3 to 7 days after surgery. Presentation typically includes headache and seizures, with altered mental status. Cerebral edema and intracranial edema are thought to be caused by impaired cerebral autoregulation of the surgically reperfused cerebral hemisphere, which is exposed postoperatively to higher cerebral perfusion and blood pressures owing to improved arterial inflow. High-grade carotid stenosis, severe bilateral carotid disease, and postoperative hypertension are major risk factors for the development of cerebral hyperperfusion syndrome. A head CT should be performed emergently to evaluate for cerebral edema and intracranial hemorrhage. Critical care treatment is focused on control of blood pressure and any seizure activity.[96]

Cranial nerve injury Most cranial nerve injuries are secondary to retraction trauma and typically resolve within 26 months; less frequently, they are the result of nerve transection. The recurrent laryngeal nerve, hypoglossal nerve, and marginal mandibular nerve are the most commonly affected. If a nerve injury is clinically suspected, phonation and swallowing should be evaluated postoperatively before the institution of oral intake. When vocal cord dysfunction is suspected, fiberoptic examination by an otolaryngologist should be completed to assess the need for further treatment.

Cardiac complications

Myocardial ischemia Carotid artery stenosis and CAD are related diseases; nearly 40% of patients undergoing CEA carry a diagnosis of symptomatic CAD.[97]

Perioperative MI is a major cause of morbidity and mortality after CEA.[98–100] Myocardial ischemia occurs in 2.0% of patients with CEA and is significantly associated with a history of hypertension and angina.[101] Symptomatic myocardial ischemia, positive serum biomarkers (troponin I or T, creatine kinase and CK-MB isoenzyme) without chest pain, and ECG changes are more common following open CEA compared with carotid artery stenting and are associated with increased mortality.[102]

Vigilance for symptoms and signs of myocardial ischemia and maintenance of adequate myocardial oxygen demand/supply balance are the basis of postoperative care.

Postoperative hypertension Postoperative hypertension is common after CEA and is related to impaired baroreceptor function as result of carotid sinus damage during dissection or its infiltration by local anesthetics. Patients with poorly controlled preoperative hypertension are at higher risk for postoperative hypertension. Severe hypertension increases the risk of bleeding, wound hematoma, and cardiac and neurologic complications, such as cerebral hyperperfusion syndrome (described previously).

Severe hypertension is an emergency and should be treated with a goal of maintaining a systolic blood pressure lower than 150 mm Hg or within 20% of preoperative values. Multiple agents are effective (labetalol, esmolol, nitroglycerine, hydralazine) and should be titrated carefully in a postanesthesia care unit or ICU setting.

Postoperative hypotension Hypotension can occur as result of hypersensitivity of the carotid sinus baroreceptor after plaque removal and usually resolves within 12 to 24 hours. Persistent hypotension can precipitate myocardial and cerebral ischemia and should be promptly treated with a combination of volume resuscitation and implementation of inotropic or alpha-agonist agents, as guided by echocardiographic and invasive hemodynamic monitoring data.

Pulmonary complications

An expanding wound hematoma may compress the trachea and cause upper airway obstruction. The airway should be expeditiously secured with an endotracheal tube, and assessment for hematoma evacuation should proceed.

Chemoreceptor dysfunction may also occur after CEA and results in hypoxemia and hypercarbia because of the reduction or absence of the normal central nervous system response mechanisms. This clinical effect is exacerbated by the use of respiratory-drive depressant drugs, like benzodiazepines and opioids.

PAD

PAD with lower extremity ischemia is a common result of generalized atherosclerosis. Functional ischemia, also known as claudication, is the result of a demand-related transient ischemia secondary to arterial stenosis. Claudication is characterized by lower extremity muscular pain and is typically induced by increased physical exertion or exercise and is relieved by rest.

Critical limb ischemia, the most severe manifestation of PAD, results from the progression of chronic atherosclerotic disease and presents with pain at rest and may present with nonhealing ulceration or gangrene on physical examination of the lower extremity. A sudden decrease in limb perfusion from an atheromatous embolism or plaque rupture with thrombosis presents more acutely with severe pain and a pale extremity with absent pulses.

Endovascular procedures (percutaneous transluminal angioplasty) and surgical bypasses (aortofemoral, femoropopliteal, and femorodistal bypass grafting) are performed to reestablish blood flow. The optimal bypass grafting technique is based on the location and morphology of the obstructive lesions, the presentation and functional status of the patients, and the preference of the vascular surgeon.[103]

Complications associated with lower limb revascularization procedures are the same as those associated with any major vascular procedure. Mortality after peripheral bypass ranges between 2% and 8% and is primarily related to myocardial ischemia.[104] Adequate pain control, continuation or initiation of beta-blockers, and administration of antiplatelet agents and a statin are essential to optimize perioperative management of these patients.

Graft thrombosis and reperfusion syndrome presenting as a compartment syndrome are specific concerns after peripheral revascularization. Hourly monitoring of the reperfused extremity is essential for early detection of compartment syndrome and urgent treatment with fasciotomy. Laboratory values should be followed for evidence of rhabdomyolysis, and patients should be kept euvolemic to minimize the risk of postoperative renal failure.

SUMMARY

Critical care management of vascular surgical patients is extremely challenging (**Box 6**). The combination of significant comorbidities in this patient population and the extensive surgical insult triggered by vascular surgery presents a high risk of severe postoperative complications. Preoperative medical risk stratification and optimization, excellent surgical technique and anesthetic management, and vigilant ICU care are integral to the successful management of patients undergoing major vascular surgery. The intensivist and critical care team must be proactive in reestablishing and maintaining physiologic homeostasis while maintaining a high index of suspicion for procedure-specific complications.

Box 6
Postoperative critical care of surgical vascular patients by major systems

Neurologic
- Multimodal pain management
- Monitoring for early signs of CVA and SCI
- Maintain appropriate CSF pressure
- Ensure adequate SCPP

Respiratory
- Early extubation when possible
- Postextubation incentive spirometry and deep-breathing maneuvers
- Lung protective ventilation strategy for ALI
- Inspiratory muscle strength training to expedite ventilator weaning process
- VAP-prevention bundle

Cardiovascular
- Monitoring for symptoms/signs of myocardial ischemia
- Check myocardial biomarkers
- Early resumption and/or starting aspirin, beta-blocker, statins
- Avoid hypertension/hypotension
- Acute limb ischemia (check peripheral pulses hourly by palpation or Doppler)
- Monitoring for limb compartment syndrome
- Daily surgical inspection of vascular surgery wounds

Renal
- Maintain euvolemia and adequate renal perfusion pressure
- Avoid nephrotoxins

Hematologic
- Monitor for bleeding complications and retroperitoneal hematoma
- Conservative blood transfusion strategy unless evidence of organ ischemia
- Thromboembolic prophylaxis

Gastrointestinal
- Monitoring for early signs of mesenteric ischemia
- Monitoring for abdominal compartment syndrome
- Early resumption of oral feeding or early starting of enteral feeding
- Stress gastritis prophylaxis

REFERENCES

1. Gopalan PD, Burrows RC. Critical care of the vascular surgery patient. Crit Care Clin 2003;19:109–25.
2. Clouse WD, Hallett JW Jr, Schaff HV, et al. Improved prognosis of thoracic aortic aneurysms: a population-based study. JAMA 1998;280:1926–9.
3. Isselbacher EM. Thoracic and abdominal aortic aneurysms. Circulation 2005;111:816–28.

4. Hiratzka LF, Bakris GL, Beckman JA, et al. 2010 ACCF/AHA/AATS/ACR/ASA/SCA/SCAI/SIR/STS/SVM guidelines for the diagnosis and management of patients with thoracic aortic disease. A report of the American College of Cardiology Foundation/American Heart Association task force on practice guidelines, American Association for Thoracic Surgery, American College of Radiology, American Stroke Association, Society of Cardiovascular Anesthesiologists, Society for Cardiovascular Angiography and Interventions, Society of Interventional Radiology, Society of Thoracic Surgeons, and Society for Vascular Medicine. J Am Coll Cardiol 2010;55:e27–129.
5. Fischbein MP, Miller DC. Long-term durability of open thoracic and thoracoabdominal aneurysm repair. Semin Vasc Surg 2009;22:74–80.
6. Conrad MF, Crawford RS, Davison JK, et al. Thoracoabdominal aneurysm repair: a 20-year perspective. Ann Thorac Surg 2007;83:S856–61.
7. Coselli JS, Bozinovski J, LeMaire SA. Open surgical repair of 2286 thoracoabdominal aortic aneurysms. Ann Thorac Surg 2007;83:S862–4.
8. Cambria RP, Clouse WD, Davison JK, et al. Thoracoabdominal aneurysm repair: results with 337 operations performed over a 15-year interval. Ann Surg 2002;236:471–9.
9. Etz CD, Di Luozzo G, Bello R, et al. Pulmonary complications after descending thoracic and thoracoabdominal aortic aneurysm repair: predictors, prevention, and treatment. Ann Thorac Surg 2007;83:S870–6.
10. Svensson LG, Hess KR, Coselli JS, et al. A prospective study of respiratory failure after high-risk surgery on the thoracoabdominal aorta. J Vasc Surg 1991;14:271–82.
11. Huynh TT, Miller CC 3rd, Estrera AL, et al. Thoracoabdominal and descending thoracic aortic aneurysm surgery in patients aged 79 years or older. J Vasc Surg 2002;36:469–75.
12. Lawrence VA, Cornell JE, Smetana GW, American College of Physicians. Strategies to reduce postoperative pulmonary complications after noncardiothoracic surgery: systematic review for the American College of Physicians. Ann Intern Med 2006;144:596–608.
13. Kindgen-Milles D, Müller E, Buhl R, et al. Nasal-continuous positive airway pressure reduces pulmonary morbidity and length of hospital stay following thoracoabdominal aortic surgery. Chest 2005;128:821–8.
14. Kashyap VS, Cambria RP, Davison JK, et al. Renal failure after thoracoabdominal aortic surgery. J Vasc Surg 1997;26:949–55.
15. Schepens MA, Defauw JJ, Hamerlijnck RP, et al. Risk assessment of acute renal failure after thoracoabdominal aortic aneurysm surgery. Ann Surg 1994;219:400–7.
16. Godet G, Fléron MH, Vicaut E, et al. Risk factors for acute postoperative renal failure in thoracic or thoracoabdominal aortic surgery: a prospective study. Anesth Analg 1997;85:1227–32.
17. Köksoy C, LeMaire SA, Curling PE, et al. Renal perfusion during thoracoabdominal aortic operations: cold crystalloid is superior to normothermic blood. Ann Thorac Surg 2002;73:730–8.
18. Lemaire SA, Jones MM, Conklin LD, et al. Randomized comparison of cold blood and cold crystalloid renal perfusion for renal protection during thoracoabdominal aortic aneurysm repair. J Vasc Surg 2009;49:11–9.
19. Sear JW. Kidney dysfunction in the postoperative period. Br J Anaesth 2005;95:20–32.
20. Coselli JS, LeMaire SA, Conklin LD, et al. Left heart bypass during descending thoracic aortic aneurysm repair does not reduce the incidence of paraplegia. Ann Thorac Surg 2004;77:1298–303.

21. Estrera AL, Miller CC 3rd, Chen EP, et al. Descending thoracic aortic aneurysm repair: 12-year experience using distal aortic perfusion and cerebrospinal fluid drainage. Ann Thorac Surg 2005;80:1290–6.
22. Svensson LG, Crawford ES, Hess KR, et al. Experience with 1509 patients undergoing thoracoabdominal aortic operations. J Vasc Surg 1993;17:357–68.
23. Huynh TT, Miller CC 3rd, Safi HJ. Delayed onset of neurologic deficit: significance and management. Semin Vasc Surg 2000;13:340–4.
24. Acher C, Wynn M. Paraplegia after thoracoabdominal aortic surgery: not just assisted circulation, hypothermic arrest, clamp and sew, or TEVAR. Ann Cardiothorac Surg 2012;1:365–72.
25. Vaughn SB, Lemaire SA, Collard CD. Case scenario: anesthetic considerations for thoracoabdominal aortic aneurysm repair. Anesthesiology 2011;115:1093–102.
26. Acher CW, Wynn M. A modern theory of paraplegia in the treatment of aneurysms of the thoracoabdominal aorta: an analysis of technique specific observed/expected ratios for paralysis. J Vasc Surg 2009;49:1117–24.
27. Griepp RB, Griepp EB. Spinal cord perfusion and protection during descending thoracic and thoracoabdominal aortic surgery: the collateral network concept. Ann Thorac Surg 2007;83:S865–9.
28. McGarvey ML, Mullen MT, Woo EY, et al. The treatment of spinal cord ischemia following thoracic endovascular aortic repair. Neurocrit Care 2007;6:35–9.
29. Ling E, Arellano R. Systematic overview of the evidence supporting the use of cerebrospinal fluid drainage in thoracoabdominal aneurysm surgery for prevention of paraplegia. Anesthesiology 2000;93:1115–22.
30. Bilal H, O'Neill B, Mahmood S, et al. Is cerebrospinal fluid drainage of benefit to neuroprotection in patients undergoing surgery on the descending thoracic aorta or thoracoabdominal aorta? Interact Cardiovasc Thorac Surg 2012;15:702–8.
31. Cinà CS, Abouzahr L, Arena GO, et al. Cerebrospinal fluid drainage to prevent paraplegia during thoracic and thoracoabdominal aortic aneurysm surgery: a systematic review and meta-analysis. J Vasc Surg 2004;40:36–44.
32. Coselli JS, LeMaire SA, Köksoy C, et al. Cerebrospinal fluid drainage reduces paraplegia after thoracoabdominal aortic aneurysm repair: results of a randomized clinical trial. J Vasc Surg 2002;35:631–9.
33. Cheung AT, Weiss SJ, McGarvey ML, et al. Interventions for reversing delayed-onset postoperative paraplegia after thoracic aortic reconstruction. Ann Thorac Surg 2002;74:413–9.
34. Hill AB, Kalman PG, Johnston KW, et al. Reversal of delayed-onset paraplegia after thoracic aortic surgery with cerebrospinal fluid drainage. J Vasc Surg 1994;20:315–7.
35. Tsusaki B, Grigore A, Cooley DA, et al. Reversal of delayed paraplegia with cerebrospinal fluid drainage after thoracoabdominal aneurysm repair. Anesth Analg 2002;94:1674.
36. Wynn MM, Mell MW, Tefera G, et al. Complications of spinal fluid drainage in thoracoabdominal aortic aneurysm repair: a report of 486 patients treated from 1987 to 2008. J Vasc Surg 2009;49:29–34.
37. Estrera AL, Sheinbaum R, Miller CC, et al. Cerebrospinal fluid drainage during thoracic aortic repair: safety and current management. Ann Thorac Surg 2009;88:9–15.
38. McGarvey ML, Cheung AT, Szeto W, et al. Management of neurologic complications of thoracic aortic surgery. J Clin Neurophysiol 2007;24:336–43.

39. Jauch EC, Saver JL, Adams HP Jr, et al. Guidelines for the early management of patients with acute ischemic stroke: a guideline for healthcare professionals from the American Heart Association/American Stroke Association. Stroke 2013;44:870–947.
40. Poldermans D, Bax JJ, Boersma E, et al. Guidelines for pre-operative cardiac risk assessment and perioperative cardiac management in non-cardiac surgery. Eur Heart J 2009;30:2769–812.
41. Kertai MD, Boersma E, Westerhout CM, et al. A combination of statins and beta-blockers is independently associated with a reduction in the incidence of perioperative mortality and nonfatal myocardial infarction in patients undergoing abdominal aortic aneurysm surgery. Eur J Vasc Endovasc Surg 2004;28:343–52.
42. Cinà CS, Clase CM. Coagulation disorders and blood product use in patients undergoing thoracoabdominal aortic aneurysm repair. Transfus Med Rev 2005;19:143–54.
43. Hardy JF, De Moerloose P, Samama M. Massive transfusion and coagulopathy: pathophysiology and implications for clinical management. Can J Anaesth 2006;53:S40–58.
44. Gertler JP, Cambria RP, Brewster DC, et al. Coagulation changes during thoracoabdominal aneurysm repair. J Vasc Surg 1996;24:936–43.
45. Levy PJ, Tabares AH, Olin JW, et al. Disseminated intravascular coagulation associated with acute ischemic hepatitis after elective aortic aneurysm repair: comparative analysis of 10 cases. J Cardiothorac Vasc Anesth 1997;11:141–8.
46. Rahe-Meyer N, Solomon C, Winterhalter M, et al. Thromboelastometry-guided administration of fibrinogen concentrate for the treatment of excessive intraoperative bleeding in thoracoabdominal aortic aneurysm surgery. J Thorac Cardiovasc Surg 2009;138:694–702.
47. Hébert PC, Wells G, Blajchman MA, et al. A multicenter, randomized, controlled clinical trial of transfusion requirements in critical care. Transfusion Requirements in Critical Care Investigators, Canadian Critical Care Trials Group. N Engl J Med 1999;340:409–17.
48. Bursi F, Barbieri A, Politi L, et al. Perioperative red blood cell transfusion and outcome in stable patients after elective major vascular surgery. Eur J Vasc Endovasc Surg 2009;37:311–8.
49. Gibbs NM, Crawford GP, Michalopoulos N. A comparison of postoperative thrombotic potential following abdominal aortic surgery, carotid endarterectomy, and femoro-popliteal bypass. Anaesth Intensive Care 1996;24:11–4.
50. Achouh PE, Madsen K, Miller CC 3rd, et al. Gastrointestinal complications after descending thoracic and thoracoabdominal aortic repairs: a 14-year experience. J Vasc Surg 2006;44:442–6.
51. Coady MA, Ikonomidis JS, Cheung AT, et al. Surgical management of descending thoracic aortic disease: open and endovascular approaches: a scientific statement from the American Heart Association. Circulation 2010;121:2780–804.
52. Bombien R, Pisimisis GT, Khoynezhad A. An update on endovascular management of acute thoracic aortic disease and future directions. Rev Cardiovasc Med 2013;14:e99–106.
53. Gutsche JT, Szeto W, Cheung AT. Endovascular stenting of thoracic aortic aneurysm. Anesthesiol Clin 2008;26:481–99.
54. Matsumura JS, Lee WA, Mitchell RS, et al. The Society for Vascular Surgery Practice guidelines: management of the left subclavian artery with thoracic endovascular aortic repair. J Vasc Surg 2009;50:1155–8.

55. Cheng D, Martin J, Shennib H, et al. Endovascular aortic repair versus open surgical repair for descending thoracic aortic disease a systematic review and meta-analysis of comparative studies. J Am Coll Cardiol 2010;55:986–1001.
56. Farber MA. Complications of endovascular aortic repair: prevention and management. Tex Heart Inst J 2009;36:444–5.
57. Nicolaou G, Ismail M, Cheng D. Thoracic endovascular aortic repair: update on indications and guidelines. Anesthesiol Clin 2013;31:451–78.
58. Ullery BW, McGarvey M, Cheung AT, et al. Vascular distribution of stroke and its relationship to perioperative mortality and neurologic outcome after thoracic endovascular aortic repair. J Vasc Surg 2012;56:1510–7.
59. Ullery BW, Cheung AT, Fairman RM, et al. Risk factors, outcomes, and clinical manifestations of spinal cord ischemia following thoracic endovascular aortic repair. J Vasc Surg 2011;54:677–84.
60. Feezor RJ, Martin TD, Hess PJ Jr, et al. Extent of aortic coverage and incidence of spinal cord ischemia after thoracic endovascular aneurysm repair. Ann Thorac Surg 2008;86:1809–14.
61. Tiesenhausen K, Amann W, Koch G, et al. Cerebrospinal fluid drainage to reverse paraplegia after endovascular thoracic aortic aneurysm repair. J Endovasc Ther 2000;7:132–5.
62. Piffaretti G, Mariscalco G, Bonardelli S, et al. Predictors and outcomes of acute kidney injury after thoracic aortic endograft repair. J Vasc Surg 2012;56:1527–34.
63. Goldfarb S, McCullough PA, McDermott J, et al. Contrast-induced acute kidney injury: specialty-specific protocols for interventional radiology, diagnostic computed tomography radiology, and interventional cardiology. Mayo Clin Proc 2009;84:170–9.
64. Cao P, De Rango P, Verzini F, et al. Endoleak after endovascular aortic repair: classification, diagnosis and management following endovascular thoracic and abdominal aortic repair. J Cardiovasc Surg 2010;51:53–69.
65. Papia G, Klein D, Lindsay TF. Intensive care of the patient following open abdominal aortic surgery. Curr Opin Crit Care 2006;12:340–5.
66. Elkouri S, Gloviczki P, McKusick MA, et al. Perioperative complications and early outcome after endovascular and open surgical repair of abdominal aortic aneurysms. J Vasc Surg 2004;39:497–505.
67. Johnson RG, Arozullah AM, Neumayer L, et al. Multivariable predictors of postoperative respiratory failure after general and vascular surgery: results from the patient safety in surgery study. J Am Coll Surg 2007;204:1188–98.
68. Calligaro KD, Azurin DJ, Dougherty MJ, et al. Pulmonary risk factors of elective abdominal aortic surgery. J Vasc Surg 1993;18:914–20.
69. Cappeller WA, Ramirez H, Kortmann H. Abdominal aortic aneurysms. Risk factors and complications and their influence on indication for operation. J Cardiovasc Surg 1989;30:572–8.
70. Markar SR, Walsh SR, Griffin K, et al. Assessment of a multifactorial risk index for predicting postoperative pneumonia after open abdominal aortic aneurysm repair. Vascular 2009;17:36–9.
71. Pathmanathan N, Beaumont N, Gratrix A. Respiratory physiotherapy in the critical care unit. Contin Educ Anaesth Crit Care Pain 2014. http://dx.doi.org/10.1093/bjaceaccp/mku005.
72. Martin AD, Smith BK, Davenport PD, et al. Inspiratory muscle strength training improves weaning outcome in failure to wean patients: a randomized trial. Crit Care 2011;15:R84.

73. Le Manach Y, Perel A, Coriat P, et al. Early and delayed myocardial infarction after abdominal aortic surgery. Anesthesiology 2005;102:885–91.
74. Chaikof EL, Brewster DC, Dalman RL, et al. The care of patients with an abdominal aortic aneurysm: the Society for Vascular Surgery practice guidelines. J Vasc Surg 2009;50:S2–49.
75. Wiesbauer F, Schlager O, Domanovits H, et al. Perioperative beta-blockers for preventing surgery-related mortality and morbidity: a systematic review and meta-analysis. Anesth Analg 2007;104:27–41.
76. Schouten O, Bax JJ, Dunkelgrun M, et al. Pro: beta-blockers are indicated for patients at risk for cardiac complications undergoing noncardiac surgery. Anesth Analg 2007;104:8–10.
77. Baxter AD, Kanji S. Protocol implementation in anesthesia: beta-blockade in non-cardiac surgery patients. Can J Anaesth 2007;54:114–23.
78. POISE Study Group. Effects of extended-release metoprolol succinate in patients undergoing non-cardiac surgery (POISE trial): a randomised controlled trial. Lancet 2008;371:1839–47.
79. Lindenauer PK, Pekow P, Wang K, et al. Perioperative beta-blocker therapy and mortality after major noncardiac surgery. N Engl J Med 2005;353:349–61.
80. Schouten O, Hoeks SE, Welten GM, et al. Effect of statin withdrawal on frequency of cardiac events after vascular surgery. Am J Cardiol 2007;100:316–20.
81. Gouëffic Y, Rozec B, Sonnard A, et al. Evidence for early nasogastric tube removal after infrarenal aortic surgery: a randomized trial. J Vasc Surg 2005;42:654–9.
82. Champagne BJ, Darling RC 3rd, Daneshmand M, et al. Outcome of aggressive surveillance colonoscopy in ruptured abdominal aortic aneurysm. J Vasc Surg 2004;39:792–6.
83. Malbrain ML, Cheatham ML, Kirkpatrick A, et al. Results from the International Conference of Experts on Intra-abdominal Hypertension and Abdominal Compartment Syndrome. I. Definitions. Intensive Care Med 2006;32:1722–32.
84. Cheatham ML, Malbrain ML, Kirkpatrick A, et al. Results from the International Conference of Experts on Intra-abdominal Hypertension and Abdominal Compartment Syndrome. II. Recommendations. Intensive Care Med 2007;33:951–62.
85. Tallgren M, Niemi T, Pöyhiä R, et al. Acute renal injury and dysfunction following elective abdominal aortic surgery. Eur J Vasc Endovasc Surg 2007;33:550–5.
86. Colson P, Ribstein J, Séguin JR, et al. Mechanisms of renal hemodynamic impairment during infrarenal aortic cross-clamping. Anesth Analg 1992;75:18–23.
87. Franks SC, Sutton AJ, Bown MJ, et al. Systematic review and meta-analysis of 12 years of endovascular abdominal aortic aneurysm repair. Eur J Vasc Endovasc Surg 2007;33:154–71.
88. Karkos CD, Harkin DW, Giannakou A, et al. Mortality after endovascular repair of ruptured abdominal aortic aneurysms: a systematic review and meta-analysis. Arch Surg 2009;144:770–8.
89. IMPROVE Trial Investigators, Powell JT, Sweeting MJ, Thompson MM, et al. Endovascular or open repair strategy for ruptured abdominal aortic aneurysm: 30 day outcomes from IMPROVE randomised trial. BMJ 2014;348:f7661.
90. Giles KA, Pomposelli F, Hamdan A, et al. Decrease in total aneurysm-related deaths in the era of endovascular aneurysm repair. J Vasc Surg 2009;49:543–50.

91. Blankensteijn JD, de Jong SE, Prinssen M, et al. Two-year outcomes after conventional or endovascular repair of abdominal aortic aneurysms. N Engl J Med 2005;352:2398–405.
92. Greenhalgh RM, Brown LC, Kwong GP, et al. Comparison of endovascular aneurysm repair with open repair in patients with abdominal aortic aneurysm (EVAR trial 1), 30-day operative mortality results: randomised controlled trial. Lancet 2004;364:843–8.
93. Litsky J, Stilp E, Njoh R, et al. Management of symptomatic carotid disease in 2014. Curr Cardiol Rep 2014;16:462.
94. Ricotta JJ, Aburahma A, Ascher E, et al. Updated Society for Vascular Surgery guidelines for management of extracranial carotid disease. J Vasc Surg 2011; 54:e1–31.
95. Allain R, Marone LK, Meltzer J, et al. Carotid endarterectomy. Int Anesthesiol Clin 2005;43:15–38.
96. Moulakakis KG, Mylonas SN, Sfyroeras GS, et al. Hyperperfusion syndrome after carotid revascularization. J Vasc Surg 2009;49:1060–8.
97. Frawley JE, Hicks RG, Horton DA, et al. Thiopental sodium cerebral protection during carotid endarterectomy: perioperative disease and death. J Vasc Surg 1994;19:732–8.
98. Estes JM, Guadagnoli E, Wolf R, et al. The impact of cardiac comorbidity after carotid endarterectomy. J Vasc Surg 1998;28:577–84.
99. Paciaroni M, Eliasziw M, Kappelle LJ, et al. Medical complications associated with carotid endarterectomy. North American Symptomatic Carotid Endarterectomy Trial (NASCET). Stroke 1999;30:1759–63.
100. Brott TG, Hobson RW 2nd, Howard G, et al. Stenting versus endarterectomy for treatment of carotid-artery stenosis. N Engl J Med 2010;363:11–23.
101. Kawahito S, Kitahata H, Tanaka K, et al. Risk factors for perioperative myocardial ischemia in carotid artery endarterectomy. J Cardiothorac Vasc Anesth 2004;18: 288–92.
102. Blackshear JL, Cutlip DE, Roubin GS, et al. Myocardial infarction after carotid stenting and endarterectomy: results from the carotid revascularization endarterectomy versus stenting trial. Circulation 2011;123:2571–8.
103. Hirsch AT, Haskal ZJ, Hertzer NR, et al. ACC/AHA 2005 Practice Guidelines for the management of patients with peripheral arterial disease (lower extremity, renal, mesenteric, and abdominal aortic): a collaborative report from the American Association for Vascular Surgery/Society for Vascular Surgery, Society for Cardiovascular Angiography and Interventions, Society for Vascular Medicine and Biology, Society of Interventional Radiology, and the ACC/AHA task force on practice guidelines (writing committee to develop guidelines for the management of patients with peripheral arterial disease): endorsed by the American Association of Cardiovascular and Pulmonary Rehabilitation; National Heart, Lung, and Blood Institute; Society for Vascular Nursing; TransAtlantic Inter-Society Consensus; and Vascular Disease Foundation. Circulation 2006;113:e463–654.
104. Nowygrod R, Egorova N, Greco G, et al. Trends, complications, and mortality in peripheral vascular surgery. J Vasc Surg 2006;43:205–16.

Index

Note: Page numbers of article titles are in **boldface** type.

Anesthesiology Clin 32 (2014) 759–770
http://dx.doi.org/10.1016/S1932-2275(14)00095-0 anesthesiology.theclinics.com

I

L

M

R

S

T

V

Printed and bound by CPI Group (UK) Ltd, Croydon, CR0 4YY
03/10/2024
01040491-0016